D1260283

THE SPECTRUM OF FACTITIOUS DISORDERS

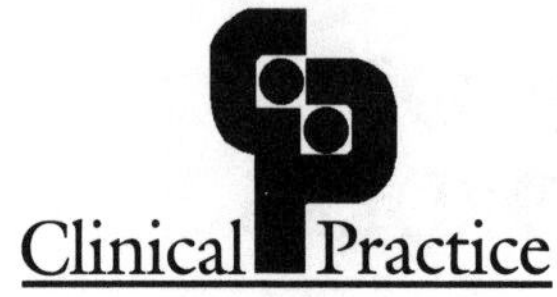

Number 40

Judith H. Gold, M.D., F.R.C.P.C.
Elissa P. Benedek, M.D.
Series Editors

THE SPECTRUM OF FACTITIOUS DISORDERS

Edited by

**Marc D. Feldman, M.D., and
Stuart J. Eisendrath, M.D.**

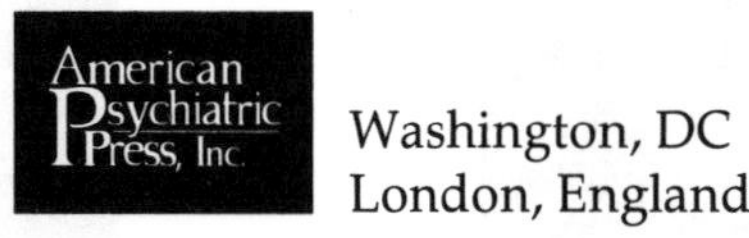

Washington, DC
London, England

Note: The authors have worked to ensure that all information in this book concerning drug dosages, schedules, and routes of administration is accurate as of the time of publication and consistent with standards set by the U.S. Food and Drug Administration and the general medical community. As medical research and practice advance, however, therapeutic standards may change. For this reason and because human and mechanical errors sometimes occur, we recommend that readers follow the advice of a physician who is directly involved in their care or the care of a member of their family.

Manufactured in the United States of America on acid-free paper
First Edition 99 98 97 96 4 3 2 1

American Psychiatric Press, Inc.
1400 K Street, N.W., Washington, DC 20005

Library of Congress Cataloging-in-Publication Data
The spectrum of factitious disorders / edited by Marc D. Feldman & Stuart J. Eisendrath.
p. cm. — (Clinical practice ; #40)
Includes bibliographical references and index.
ISBN 0-88048-909-X (cloth)
1. Factitious disorders. I. Feldman, Marc D., 1958– . II. Eisendrath, Stuart J., 1948– . III. Series: Clinical practice ; no. 40.
[DNLM: 1. Factitious Disorders. W1 CL767J no. 40 1996 / WM 178 S741 1996]
RC569.5.F27S67 1996
616.89—dc20
DNLM/DLC
for Library of Congress 96-13799
CIP

British Library Cataloguing in Publication Data
A CIP record is available from the British Library.

To Jackie, Lee, and Sara

To Debra, Adam, and Allison

Contents

Contributors

Stuart J. Eisendrath, M.D.
Professor of Clinical Psychiatry, the University of California, San Francisco School of Medicine; Director, Consultation-Liaison Program, the University of California, San Francisco Medical Center, San Francisco, California

Adriana Feder, M.D.
Assistant Clinical Professor of Psychiatry at the University of California, San Francisco. Assistant Director of the Psychiatric Consultation-Liaison Program at Moffitt-Long Hospitals

Marc D. Feldman, M.D.
Associate Professor, Vice Chair for Clinical Services, and Director of the Division of Adult Psychiatry in the Department of Psychiatry and Behavioral Neurobiology at the University of Alabama, Birmingham (UAB); Medical Director, the UAB Center for Psychiatric Medicine; Regional Medical Director, United Behavioral Systems, Inc.

Charles V. Ford, M.D.
Professor of Psychiatry and Director of the Neuropsychiatry Clinic of the Department of Psychiatry and Behavioral Neurobiology at the University of Alabama at Birmingham

Don R. Lipsitt, M.D.
Clinical Professor of Psychiatry at Harvard Medical School and Chair of the Department of Psychiatry at Mount Auburn Hospital, Cambridge, Massachusetts. Editor-in-Chief, *General Hospital Psychiatry,* and member of the Boston Psychoanalytic Society and Institute

Theodore Nadelson, M.D.
Clinical Professor of Psychiatry at Boston University School of Medicine, Boston, Massachusetts

Barbara M. Ostfeld, Ph.D.
Clinical Professor of Pediatrics and Clinical Associate Professor of Psychiatry at the Robert Wood Johnson Medical School of the University of Medicine and Dentistry of New Jersey, New Brunswick, New Jersey; Director of Pediatric Psychology at St. Peter's Medical Center and Associate Director of the New Jersey State Sudden Infant Death Syndrome Resource Center, New Brunswick, New Jersey; Former Chair of the Munchausen Syndrome by Proxy Education Committee of the National Association of Apnea Professionals

Pamela E. Parker, M.D.
Assistant Professor of Psychiatry at the University of Alabama School of Medicine, Tuscaloosa; former Director of Consultation Psychiatry at the University of Alabama School of Medicine at Birmingham

Deirdre Conway Rand, Ph.D.
Psychologist in private practice with a dual emphasis on clinical and forensic work, Mill Valley, California

Roxenne Smith, M.A.
Professional writer and gerontologist, Ozona, Florida

Beatrice Crofts Yorker, J.D., R.N., M.S.
Associate Provost for Faculty Relations and Associate Professor of Nursing at Georgia State University, Atlanta, Georgia; clinical specialist in child and adolescent psychiatric nursing, and attorney; Fellow of the American Academy of Nursing

Introduction
to the Clinical Practice Series

Over the years of its existence the series of monographs entitled *Clinical Insights* gradually became focused on providing current, factual, and theoretical material of interest to the clinician working outside of a hospital setting. To reflect this orientation, the name of the Series has been changed to *Clinical Practice.*

The Clinical Practice Series will provide books that give the mental health clinician a practical, clinical approach to a variety of psychiatric problems. These books will provide up-to-date literature reviews and emphasize the most recent treatment methods. Thus, the publications in the Series will interest clinicians working both in psychiatry and in the other mental health professions.

Each year a number of books will be published dealing with all aspects of clinical practice. In addition, from time to time when appropriate, the publications may be revised and updated. Thus, the Series will provide quick access to relevant and important areas of psychiatric practice. Some books in the Series will be authored by a person considered to be an expert in that particular area; others will be edited by such an expert, who will also draw together other knowledgeable authors to produce a comprehensive overview of that topic.

Some of the books in the Clinical Practice Series will have their foundation in presentations at an annual meeting of the American Psychiatric Association. All will contain the most recently available information on the subjects discussed. Theoretical and scientific data will be applied to clinical situations, and case illustrations will be utilized in order to make the material even more relevant for the practitioner. Thus, the Clinical Practice Series should provide educational reading in a compact format especially designed for the mental health clinician–psychiatrist.

Judith H. Gold, M.D., F.R.C.P.C.
Series Editor
Clincal Practice Series

Clinical Practice Series Titles

The Spectrum of Factitious Disorders (#40)
Edited by Marc D. Feldman, M.D., and Stuart J. Eisendrath, M.D.

Group Therapy for Schizophrenic Patients (#39)
By Nick Kanas, M.D.

Sexual Harassment in the Workplace and Academia: Psychiatric Issues (#38)
Edited by Diane K. Shrier, M.D.

Use of Neuroleptics in Children (#37)
Edited by Mary Ann Richardson, Ph.D., and Gary Haugland, M.A.

The New Pharmacotherapy of Schizophrenia (#36)
Edited by Alan Breier, M.D.

Clinical Assessment and Management of Severe Personality Disorders (#35)
Edited by Paul S. Links, M.D., M.Sc., F.R.C.P.C.

Predictors of Treatment Response in Mood Disorders (#34)
Edited by Paul J. Goodnick, M.D.

Successful Psychiatric Practice in Changing Times: Current Dilemmas, Choices, and Solutions (#33)
Edited by Edward K. Silberman, M.D.

Alternatives to Hospitalization for Acute Psychiatric Treatment (#32)
Edited by Richard Warner, M.B., D.P.M.

Behavioral Complications in Alzheimer's Disease (#31)
Edited by Brian A. Lawlor, M.D.

Patient Violence and the Clinician (#30)
Edited by Burr S. Eichelman, M.D., Ph.D., and Anne C. Hartwig, J.D., Ph.D.

Effective Use of Group Therapy in Managed Care (#29)
Edited by K. Roy MacKenzie, M.D., F.R.C.P.C.

Rediscovering Childhood Trauma: Historical Casebook and Clinical Applications (#28)
Edited by Jean M. Goodwin, M.D., M.P.H.

Treatment of Adult Survivors of Incest (#27)
Edited by Patricia L. Paddison, M.D.

Madness and Loss of Motherhood: Sexuality, Reproduction, and Long-Term Mental Illness (#26)
Edited by Roberta J. Apfel, M.D., M.P.H., and Maryellen H. Handel, Ph.D.

Psychiatric Aspects of Symptom Management in Cancer Patients (#25)
Edited by William Breitbart, M.D., and Jimmie C. Holland, M.D.

Responding to Disaster: A Guide for Mental Health Professionals (#24)
Edited by Linda S. Austin, M.D.

Psychopharmacological Treatment Complications in the Elderly (#23)
Edited by Charles A. Shamoian, M.D., Ph.D.

Anxiety Disorders in Children and Adolescents (#22)
By Syed Arshad Husain, M.D., F.R.C.P.C., F.R.C.Psych., and Javad Kashani, M.D.

Suicide and Clinical Practice (#21)
Edited by Douglas Jacobs, M.D.

Special Problems in Managing Eating Disorders (#20)
Edited by Joel Yager, M.D., Harry E. Gwirtsman, M.D., and Carole K. Edelstein, M.D.

Children and AIDS (#19)
Edited by Margaret L. Stuber, M.D.

Current Treatments of Obsessive-Compulsive Disorder (#18)
Edited by Michele Tortora Pato, M.D., and Joseph Zohar, M.D.

Benzodiazepines in Clinical Practice: Risks and Benefits (#17)
Edited by Peter P. Roy-Byrne, M.D., and Deborah S. Cowley, M.D.

Adolescent Psychotherapy (#16)
Edited by Marcia Slomowitz, M.D.

Family Approaches in Treatment of Eating Disorders (#15)
Edited by D. Blake Woodside, M.D., M.Sc., F.R.C.P.C., and Lorie Shekter-Wolfson, M.S.W., C.S.W.

Clinical Management of Gender Identity Disorders in Children and Adults (#14)
Edited by Ray Blanchard, Ph.D., and Betty W. Steiner, M.B., F.R.C.P.C.

New Perspectives on Narcissism (#13)
Edited by Eric M. Plakun, M.D.

The Psychosocial Impact of Job Loss (#12)
By Nick Kates, M.B.B.S., F.R.C.P.C., Barrie S. Greiff, M.D., and Duane Q. Hagen, M.D.

Office Treatment of Schizophrenia (#11)
Edited by Mary V. Seeman, M.D., F.R.C.P.C., and Stanley E. Greben, M.D., F.R.C.P.C.

Psychiatric Care of Migrants: A Clinical Guide (#10)
By Joseph Westermeyer, M.D., M.P.H., Ph.D.

Family Involvement in Treatment of the Frail Elderly (#9)
Edited by Marion Zucker Goldstein, M.D.

Measuring Mental Illness: Psychometric Assessment for Clinicians (#8)
Edited by Scott Wetzler, Ph.D.

Juvenile Homicide (#7)
Edited by Elissa P. Benedek, M.D., and Dewey G. Cornell, Ph.D.

The Neuroleptic Malignant Syndrome and Related Conditions (#6)
By Arthur Lazarus, M.D., Stephan C. Mann, M.D., and Stanley N. Caroff, M.D.

Anxiety: New Findings for the Clinician (#5)
Edited by Peter Roy-Byrne, M.D.

Anxiety and Depressive Disorders in the Medical Patient (#4)
By Leonard R. Derogatis, Ph.D., and Thomas N. Wise, M.D.

Family Violence: Emerging Issues of a National Crisis (#3)
Edited by Leah J. Dickstein, M.D., and Carol C. Nadelson, M.D.

Divorce as a Developmental Process (#2)
Edited by Judith H. Gold, M.D., F.R.C.P.C.

Treating Chronically Mentally Ill Women (#1)
Edited by Leona L. Bachrach, Ph.D., and Carol C. Nadelson, M.D.

Acknowledgments

We wish to express our appreciation to the authors whose work appears in this volume. Each was enthusiastic about contributing to this, the first text for professionals that is devoted to factitious disorders, and we value the expertise and collegiality they brought to the project.

Marci Miller, A.R.N.P., M.S., offered important insights into the toll on nurses in Chapter 10, titled "Personal and Interpersonal Toll of Factitious Disorders." Cheryl L. Wilke, J.D., Joel H. Feldman, J.D., and David B. Allen, R.N., J.D., assisted in compiling and cross checking the legal references. Many thanks.

We appreciate the professionalism of our publisher, American Psychiatric Press. We also want to extend our sincere thanks to Judith H. Gold, M.D., F.R.C.P.C., Editor of the Clinical Practice Series, who suggested that we embark upon this project and gave us her warm support.

Finally, we want to thank our administrative and secretarial staffs, including Jacquelyn Boswell, Tammy Harbin, Pam Armstrong, and Yvonne Waldon.

Introduction

Don R. Lipsitt, M.D.

> The construction of fictions—of various degrees of falsity—to ease our path occasionally, to repair a faltering relation, is one of the functions of imagination, and we should do well to be in no hurry to despise imagination, upon which we are also dependent, after all, for the construction of nonfictions, which we can hardly do without.
>
> Leslie Farber,
> *Lying, Despair, Jealousy, Envy, Sex, Suicide, and the Good Life*

The line between truth and fiction is sometimes perilously thin. It is on the basis of ability to perceive the difference that we often judge a person to be in or out of touch with reality. Our criteria for declaring an individual psychotic are reasonably clear, but when we begin to impute willfulness to disease we tread on uncertain ground. Relegating motive to the unconscious broadens our tolerance of "antisocial" behavior and permits some degree of distinction between disease and deception. Our empathy swells in the presence of one believed to be victimized by disease but virtually evaporates at a hint that we may be the victims of a deceiver. The diagnosis of factitious disorder often hinges upon who is the deceiver and who is the deceived.

The Purloined Sick Role

In all likelihood, factitious disorder is both disease and deception, presenting one of the most challenging (and potentially vexing) variants of psychopathology in medical experience. If we impute a conscious motive to the wish to be sick, we regard this as strange behavior indeed; only in the case of the true malingerer, whose behavior is quite transparently designed for some personal gain, does logic prevail. If we can detect no reason for such a desire, our preference is to assume that there must be strong propulsion from deeply unconscious and complex roots.

Such behavior lies outside the parameters of the "sick role" as defined by Talcott Parsons (1951). In this role, sick individuals are excused from social responsibility, are expected to perceive their condition as undesirable, lack voluntary control over it and therefore are not considered at fault, and are expected to seek competent help in ameliorating or curing the condition. But patients who would feign illness merely for the sake of being patients would appear, in the words of Susan Sontag (1977), to prefer to dwell in the "kingdom of the sick" rather than the "kingdom of the well" (p. 3). In the sociologic realm of illness behavior, those patients who fulfill the criteria of the Parsonian sick role are considered "good" patients and those who utilize it fraudulently are considered "bad." The concept of "abnormal illness behavior" (Mechanic 1963; Pilowsky 1969), although conceptualized in application to individuals with more or less bona fide illness, can be extended emphatically to the voluntary induction of illness, whether for primary or secondary gain.

It is a memorable event when a physician has been "snookered" by the patient with factitious disorder. Detection may be immediate or, perhaps more often, delayed. The more distant one becomes from the original encounter, the more embarrassment may ensue from the "missed diagnosis." Most physicians have seen at least one such patient in their careers, although recognition may be late or never occur.

Complex Psychodynamics

The complex determinants of the patient's ruse are as much a mystery as the causes of cancer or the common cold. Partly, our ignorance stems from the evasiveness of these patients, who habitually sign out or "disappear" only to reappear again elsewhere. Such behavior provides us with little opportunity to study the phenomenon. While a few patients with factitious disorder have agreed to a course of psychotherapy, most often the therapy provides only a short sabbatical from their profession of illness.

Most of what we assume to be true about the dynamics of medical deception is based entirely upon conjecture. We know from clinical experience and human awareness that lying usually is intended to protect secrets and avoid anxiety (Ford 1996). What secrets are being guarded against we must usually infer from the scant factual data accessible to us. The shallowness of the patient's responses to searching questions and the gaps in what initially appears to be a coherent history raise our index of suspicion. We know that these patients make us angry, and we are inclined to retaliate, even while maintaining professional restraint. We infer a basic sadomasochistic style of interpersonal behavior. Some physicians, in a kind of "countercreative" revenge, will attempt to match wits with these individuals who demonstrate sometimes extraordinary cunning and innovation. In so doing, the physician likewise adopts a bit of a Munchausenian stance, attempting to devise ways to outfox the faux.

Fictitious Factitia

There is even a touch of the fable in the history of the origin of Munchausen syndrome. The Baron's stories were patently transparent fantasies, with only entertainment and no deception intended. They had no medical content and involved no convoluted perigrinating. In fact, as Nadelson points out in Chapter 1, the so-called adventures of Baron von Münchhausen were not even written by him. Instead, they were written by an impecunious liar, cheat, and embezzler who appropriated the stories and penned them in England (not Germany) for personal profit (Raspe 1948). The terms *lying* and *Munchausen* were inextricably linked in German culture when fibbing children were called "little Munchausens." But the formal connection between Münchausen's fables and the pseudologia fantastica of factitious illness was established by a physician, Dr. Richard Asher, who in 1951 named the disorder *Munchausen's syndrome* (Asher 1951).

Meaning From Suffering

We can assume that people who choose illness as a way of life might be attempting to derive some kind of meaning out of suffering, presumably suffering that has stemmed from early life experience, various kinds of trauma, hospitalizations, and family dysfunction. For example, a woman reared in squalor by an inadequate mother of seven children and an abusive, jail-guard father seemingly began her chronic Munchausen behavior after hospitalization for a relatively minor accident (Lipsitt 1986). Factitious disorder is not the only disorder that is cultivated in this etiologic soil; the potential for virtually every pathologic entity is said to be heightened by early deprivation and emotional trauma. To the extent that patients are incapable consciously of relating their current behaviors to past events, others, including physicians, are invited to become their caretakers and interpreters of their symptoms. Entering the sick role by design is a desperate way of trying to communicate. Using the body for this function is not so unusual as it might seem: conversion disorder, somatization, and hypochondriasis are other examples. Indeed, the patient presenting to the emergency room with authentic chest pain may not be conscious of the possible etiologies he or she invites the physician to explore. But the patient with factitious disorder abuses the sick role. He or she misuses the doctor-patient relationship for surreptitious, perhaps unconscious gain, although the contrived symptoms would appear to be conscious. As described in Chapters 2 and 3, it is perhaps this ratio of conscious to unconscious elements in such illness behavior that determines whether a particular instance of factitious disorder is an illness or a deception.

Presenting one's illness to others, especially physicians, usually revolves around efforts to sustain integrity of the self, whether psychological or bodily. Keeping truth from others is not only self-protective but also an act of revenge for past hurts and exploitation by others, a way of "doing unto others what they have done unto me." Keeping truth from others is largely conscious, but keeping truth from oneself is very likely unconscious, a way of protecting a fragile identity. Being a "professional patient" is no small task, and its successful negotiation cloaks one in a unique identity. Imposturing patients may even be the objects of some admiration in the way that magicians are revered for their capacity to fool us, while making fools of us. In that context, Greenacre (1958) has hypothesized that the victims are at least in part enablers of the behavior of impostors.

The patient with factitious disorder, like the fetishist, protects the self from the anxiety caused by awareness of a bit of traumatic reality, just as the individual with paraphilia covets objects that offer "reassurance" that the woman "really" does have a penis. Both the fetishist and the factitial patient say in essence, "If I can make up a story that is believable when I know it to be false, then maybe what I know to be really the truth cannot be believed." Schreier (1992) suggests that factitious disorder by proxy (also called *Munchausen syndrome by proxy*) may be such a form of "character perversion," in which a self-doubting mother "assures" herself (and others) of her goodness by inflicting harm upon her own child. Perhaps the simulating patient detoxifies the painful reality of his or her past by inventing a falsity that even he or she comes to believe. By their risky, but paradoxically self-preserving, antics, these individuals assume notoriety, even immortality and a kind of professional acclaim through such eponymous identities as the Indiana Cyclone, the Duncan Hines of Hospitals, the Gasoline Injector, and the Red Baron or Baroness. Some of these people appear in the professional literature more often than aspiring academics.

Risking Life to Survive

These patients are not only magicians; they are high-wire acrobats, always living on the edge of disaster. In giving up a little bit of themselves, they preserve what remains and, in a sense, make the whole even greater. This reminds us of Menninger's concept of partial suicide (Menninger 1934), a process similar to animal autotomy in which a piece of the body is sacrificed to a limb-capturing trap in the service of self-preservation. At the same time, these chameleon-like individuals can shift effortlessly from active to passive, playing the roles alternately of victim or victimizer—or, as in Simmel's (1926) description of the "doctor game" of childhood, playing at one time the patient and at another the doctor. The child, in fantasy, gets to be both mother and father, alternating between hurting and being hurt in a child's symbolic perception of parental lovemaking. This capacity to vacillate from caretaker to care-receiver is seen in the extreme in the behavior of the mother in representative cases of factitious disorder by proxy (Meadow 1977). Paradoxically, she harms her children in order to seem to be a "better" mother; simultaneously, she enlists extensive solicitous caring for herself, at least briefly. Attempts to understand the phenomenology, dynamics, and management of the bizarre interaction between perpetrator and victim in factitious disorder by proxy are considered more fully in Chapters 6 through 9. Early recognition and prompt intervention can be life-saving for the child and potentially therapeutic for the mother.

One author, describing Munchausen syndrome itself, says that the patient performs as though all the world is a stage in some kind of theater of the absurd (Spiro 1968). The "pretend" nature of the performance seems to proclaim that "as long as I know I am pretending I am sick, then I know that I am really alive and well," a modification of Sholem Aleichem's remark that "as long as my teeth are chattering, I know I'm alive." However, the Nietzschean proverb that "that which does not kill me makes me stronger" is not borne out in the patients with Munchausen syndrome who have actually been maimed or permanently disabled as a result of their impostures.

Sexual Pleasure in Illness

The greater the deception, the greater the personal gain from the dissimulator's point of view, a self-deception described with uncanny insight by Thomas Mann (1969) in *Confessions of Felix Krull, Confidence Man.* Having duped his mother into believing him ill, young Felix reports that

> [s]he looked at me with a growing sense of reality. . . . Starting up in bed with a fitful, shuddering motion, I drew my basin toward me and bent over it with spasmodic twitchings and contortions of my whole body, such as no one could witness without profound emotion. . . . [T]hen I launched upon my main effort, a prolonged attack of cramps and retching which made it seem that I would never breathe again. My mother held my head. . . . By the time my limbs finally began to relax she was quite overcome and, exclaiming "I'll send for Dusing!" she rushed out of the room. I sank back among the pillows exhausted but full of indescribable joy and satisfaction. . . . I had produced these symptoms as effectively as though I had nothing to do with their

> appearance . . . out of nothing more than imagination and the daring exploitation of [my] own body. . . . [O]nly he who has succeeded in creating a compelling and effective reality out of nothing, out of sheer inward knowledge and contemplation—in short, out of nothing more than imagination and the daring exploitation of his own body . . . understands the strange and dreamlike satisfaction with which I rested from my creative task. (pp. 33–34)

The sexualized nature of the feigned illness, often ascribed to the behavior of the Munchausen patient, is here unmistakable. Felix goes on:

> I was highly excited; I had concentrated my whole being upon an act of will; I was drunk with the intensity of my own performance in my role of parodying nature—a performance that had to be masterly if it was not to be ridiculous; I was delirious with the alternate tension and relaxation necessary to give reality, in my own eyes and others, to a condition that did not exist. . . ." (p. 37)

The deception further elaborates the oedipal drama by demeaning the all-knowing father-physician-authority (the family physician, Dr. Dusing), an aggressive act to which Felix makes mother an unwitting accomplice. He says,

> Indeed, the medical profession is not different from any other; its members are, for the most part, ordinary empty-headed dolts, ready to see what is not there and to deny the obvious. Any untrained person, if he is a connoisseur and lover of the body, exceeds them in this knowledge of its subtler mysteries and can easily lead them around by the nose. (p. 36)

Does Felix Krull have a disorder, an illness? Is his way of resolving oedipal conflict less respectable than a conversion disorder or other attempts at compromise formation that we call illnesses? Are we not in the dark about the whole process of symptom or illness "selection"? Is the use of terms such as *crock, turkey, Munchausen syndrome,* and others—maybe even borderline and sociopath—at least partly determined by the decrement in our own self-esteem when we attempt to understand and to treat those individuals who frustrate our honest efforts?

The complex dynamics of the perpetrator of feigned illness were revealed to me by a man who, as an adolescent, had faked belly pain in order to avoid school for a day. His father, with whom he had a very distant and disappointing relationship, became concerned and took his son to the doctor, who diagnosed appendicitis. The boy knew he did not have appendicitis but acquiesced to surgery nonetheless. By so doing, he not only encouraged his father's interest and compassion but also believed he would establish a lasting alliance with his father, who he knew had a great disdain for doctors. The boy was certain that his father would be reinforced in his attitudes toward physicians when he learned of the diagnostic and therapeutic error; his fantasy was that he and father together had shown the doctor to be a fool. He imagined also that this collaborative achievement would save him from the wrath he could expect from his father had he stopped only at the point of having faked his pain to stay home from school.

Ethics of Detection

It would seem that ethical dilemmas in working with all factitious disorders (see Chapter 4) should be resolved essentially on the basis of the principle of "first, do no harm," which is applied in most medical situations. They should not be derived from anger and frustration, resulting in the posting or distribution of "black lists" or "rogues' galleries" of culpable patients. Room searches, surreptitious record procurement and phone calls, and covert surveillance should be for the purpose of protecting factitious patients from themselves, children from their disordered mothers, or society from the wasting of scarce medical resources and—in the type of case discussed in Chapter 5—the misappropriation of mechanisms for legal redress. These techniques should not be used simply to establish our reputations as medical detectives. Overall, the principles of caring for both suicidal and homicidal patients would seem to apply, even in the absence of an established doctor-patient relationship. Perhaps one of the most difficult ethical questions is when to separate, and possibly reunite, mother and child in suspected factitious disorder by proxy, and this issue is considered in detail in Chapters 6 and 7.

Prospects for Treatment

As for treatment of factitious disorders, we are still at something of a loss. For the most part, attempts to influence the behavior have been unsuccessful. No doubt, some of the patients who fall on Nadelson's scale closer to the "normal"range (Nadelson 1979; see also Chapter 1 in this volume) may benefit from therapeutic intervention, but those with more extreme presentations seem extraordinarily refractory. At the very least, they would merit the designation of "negative therapeutic reaction," Freud's characterization of patients whose every fiber resisted the psychoanalyst's efforts. At worst, they may be said to be continually "gaming the system" when they acquiesce to a course of psychiatric treatment, only to move on soon thereafter to the next state or city, seeking hospital admission for another fantastic illness.

In Chapter 10, Feldman and Smith use first-person accounts to illustrate the intense feelings mobilized in friends, family members, caregivers, and patients themselves as factitious disorders play out. Eisendrath and Feder's management approach, described in Chapter 11, can be commended for its humanity, its tact, and its respect for the patient no matter the symptomatology. No less should be available to any patient, provided we can tolerate the disappointment (and perhaps anger) that may ensue. Just as we learn to work with "objectionable" patients with borderline or narcissistic disorders, we may be able to learn to work with factitious patients, even those referred to as having Munchausen syndrome. The chapters in this volume carry us further in search of that objective. They stress the need to treat with acceptance and understanding these patients with bizarre behavioral disorders. In so doing, we will take heed of Farber's cautionary advice to "be in no hurry to despise imagination."

References

Asher R: Munchausen's syndrome. Lancet 1:339–341, 1951

Farber LH: Lying, Despair, Jealousy, Envy, Sex, Suicide, and the Good Life. New York, Basic Books, 1976, p 218

Ford CV: Lies! Lies!! Lies!!! The Psychology of Deceit. Washington, DC, American Psychiatric Press, 1996, pp 23–46

Greenacre P: The imposter. Psychoanal Q 27:359–382, 1958

Lipsitt DR: The factitious patient who sues (letter). Am J Psychiatry 143:1482, 1986

Mann T: Confessions of Felix Krull, Confidence Man. New York, Vintage Books, 1969

Meadow R: Munchausen syndrome by proxy: the hinterland of child abuse. Lancet 2:343–345, 1977

Mechanic D: Some implications of illness behavior for medical sampling. N Engl J Med 269:244–247, 1963

Menninger KA: Polysurgery and polysurgical addiction. Psychoanal Q 3:173–199, 1934

Nadelson T: The Munchausen spectrum: borderline character features. Gen Hosp Psychiatry 1:11–17, 1979

Parsons T: The Social System. Glencoe, Free Press, 1951

Pilowsky I: Abnormal illness behavior. Br J Med Psychol 42:347–351, 1969

Raspe RE: The Singular Travels, Campaigns, and Adventures of Baron Munchausen. London, Cresset Press, 1948

Schreier HA: Munchausen syndrome by proxy. Bull Menninger Clin 56:421–437, 1992

Simmel E: The "doctor game," illness and the profession of medicine. Int J Psychoanal 7:470–483, 1926

Sontag S: Illness as Metaphor. New York, Farrar, Strauss and Giroux, 1977

Spiro HR: Chronic factitious illness. Arch Gen Psychiatry 18:569–579, 1968

CHAPTER 1

Historical Perspectives on the Spectrum of Sickness

From "Crock" to "Crook"

Theodore Nadelson, M.D.

Most physicians informally group their patients' somatic complaints. In one category are "real" symptoms; the symptoms the patients report clearly derive from anatomic or physiologic disturbances. In the other category are symptoms that appear more murky and emotionally colored. The move within the field of psychiatry toward greater objectivity and rigor in diagnosis has led increasingly to sharply defined, validated criteria for psychological entities. However, with the refinement of these definitions, some discontinuity remains among the various diagnoses subsumed by the DSM-IV heading, "Somatoform Disorders" (American Psychiatric Association 1994). In this chapter, the author develops a plan for linking the concepts associated with abnormal illness behavior. Housed in its own section of DSM-IV, Factitious Disorders, the central subject of this book, similarly lacks clear connections to the other forms of abnormal illness behavior.

A Synthesis of Categories

Presented here is a synthesis of "common sense" ideas regarding sickness and the formal psychiatric diagnoses in which somatization occurs. The resulting spectrum is intended not only to interconnect the somatoform disorder diagnoses found in DSM-IV but also to integrate understanding of the relationship between the "real" and the "psychiatric" or the "factitial." These categorizations will be further elucidated later. This schema has proved helpful to both psychiatric and nonpsychiatric clinicians by bringing into clearer focus the confusing confluence of a particular patient's personal responsibility and unconscious motivation. It also has been helpful in instructing students of medicine and other health care providers; most health care education focuses on the patient who has had no part in the etiology of the illness and who, at the very least, wishes to get better as soon as possible. This type of patient is presented as a Group A patient within this chapter (see Table 1–1).

Other kinds of patients are usually designated as psychiatric. Yet even when such patients do receive a confirmatory psychiatric diagnosis, this recognition of an authentic mental disorder never completely deflects pejoratives such as "crock" (Lipsitt 1970) when nonpsychiatric clinicians refer to such patients. Although many patients present with physical symptoms colored, at least in part, by emotions (Ford 1983; Hoeper et al. 1980; Voiss 1995), the motivations of somatizing patients with psychiatric diagnoses are still generally viewed with suspicion by the public (e.g., the friends and families) and by their nonpsychiatric physicians.

It may be helpful to start at the end of the spectrum usually seen as isolated from the rest of medicine, characterized by the patient presenting with factitial symptoms and signs. Whereas somatic expressions of psychological problems are usually seen as part of sickness and deserving of medical care, mimicry of disease violates the boundary of the patient role. Examination of the most chronic and extreme form of factitious disorder, namely Munchausen syndrome, may better inform us of the more familiar presentations as well.

False Patients: Factitious Disorder and Munchausen Syndrome

Factitious somatic disease has always been separated from the rest of medical practice because patients with factitial maladies

Table 1–1. The spectrum of somatic presentation: real "patients" to "crocks" and "crooks"

Sickness assignment	Medical category A	Psychiatric category B	Legal category C-1	Legal category C-2
General diagnostic groupings	Infection, trauma, metabolic disease, cancer	**Somatoform disorders** Somatization disorder Undifferentiated somatoform conversion disorder Body dysmorphic disorder Pain disorder Hypochondriasis Somatoform disease NOS	**Factitious disorders** Prototypical factitious disorder Munchausen syndrome	Malingering
Character diagnosis	Not relevant	Various (neurotic, character disorder, alexithymic)	Borderline personality	Borderline or antisocial
View of specificity	Assumed specificity	Psychological mechanisms presented as etiology		Fraud
Reason for medical poblem	"Accident"; patient as victim	Sensitive to emotional stress; diathesis — Abnormal illness behavior; expression of severe psychopathology		Personal gain

(continued)

Table 1–1. The spectrum of somatic presentation: real "patients" to "crocks" and "crooks" *(continued)*

Sickness assignment	**Medical category A**	**Psychiatric category B**	**Legal category C-1**	**Legal category C-2**
Physician's attitude toward patient	"This is a real patient, a legitimate victim"	"This is a psychiatric patient, a crock, but still a patient"	"This is a false patient, not a patient"	"This is a crook"
Patient role	Afflicted	Welcoming sickness; care-eliciting behavior	Causing sickness; care-coercing behavior	Fraud
Sickness source as viewed by physician	"Body"	"Mind"	"Character"	
Sickness source as viewed by patient	Body	Body	Confused	Self
Goal of most caretakers	Cure, manage, palliate	Stabilize, manage, cure	Neutralize, help	Reveal fraud, punish

Note. NOS = not otherwise specified.

1) feign or produce their own disease, 2) are aware of their role in the deception (although their underlying motivation for putting themselves at risk is probably unconscious), and 3) keep their simulation or induction of illness secret.

In Asher's (1951) report in which the Munchausen designation was first applied to chronic factitial behavior, Asher described "a common syndrome which most doctors have seen, but about which little has been written." Patients who falsify disease were arrayed, somewhat facetiously, under ponderous Latin subheadings (e.g., *laparotomophilia migrans*) on the basis of the organ system chosen for simulation. Abdominal, hemorrhagic, and neurologic types were distinguished. The levity within Asher's report cloaked a darker picture of personal suffering and cost to the health care system.

In a stroke of creativity, Asher borrowed the term *Munchausen syndrome* from Rudolph Erich Raspe, an eighteenth century courtier and author of children's books. Raspe had been the first to usurp the name of a real, living German cavalry officer, Baron Karl Friedrich Hieronymus von Münchhausen (1720–1797), recreating him in his 1785 pamphlet, "Baron Munchausen's Narrative of his Marvelous Travels and Campaigns in Russia," as an amusing fictional character who always lied, albeit harmlessly. Raspe's book was an immediate financial success, and it depicted the baron as preoccupied with tales of his own heroic military conquests and miraculous escapes from foreign dungeons (Luce 1978). In reality, there is no evidence to suggest that the baron had a history of lying in order to deceive others; instead, Raspe exercised considerable literary license. Nonetheless, Asher continued the notion of a truth-bending "Munchausen" when he "respectfully dedicated the syndrome [of medical deception] to him." The term *Munchausen syndrome* has lived in perpetuity with more fame than could be expected for an otherwise middling German nobleman.

Asher loosely characterized the psychological attributes of patients with Munchausen syndrome as those of "hysterics, schizophrenics, masochists or psychopaths of some kind." These patients continue to be noted in all writing on the subject as "wanderers," with their destinations being doctors' offices, clinics, and hospitals. The Munchausen patient's rootlessness and frequency of false presentation of disease led to coining of the term *hospital hoboes* (Clark and Melnick 1958). Despite its greater descriptive accuracy, it has not gained the popularity of the initial eponymous reference.

Patients with full-blown Munchausen syndrome represent a small subset, perhaps 10% (Reich and Gottfried 1983), of all patients with factitious disorders, however. The remaining group includes patients who imitate or self-induce disease to a lesser extent and only episodically. This group of factitious disorder patients consists mostly of women who often hold responsible jobs, generally within medical settings (Nadelson 1979). Individuals with Munchausen syndrome can become concerned, however, when their behavior—which can appear addictive in quality—comes close to endangering their employment or health. The following case is offered as an illustration.

Case 1

A telephone caller identified herself as a nurse and requested reprints on factitious disease as well as consultation time with the writer. When asked if her purpose was research, she replied that she wanted psychiatric help. She had planned to come to Boston. "I have an addiction," she said, "and I'm planning on checking into the MGH [Massachusetts General Hospital]. In the Midwest," she continued, "I'm known as the 'Baroness.'" The caller revealed that she had recently self-induced a unilateral ophthalmoplegia, almost eventuating in a surgical procedure. After that "close call" she recognized her desperate need for psychiatric help.

There is continued clinical reporting of illness falsification, and clearly the type and magnitude of the deceptions are limited only by the patient's creativity (Aduan et al. 1979; Baile et al. 1992; Folks and Kinney 1992; Reich and Gottfried 1983). A review of the multiplicity of ways in which such patients can present is impossible because of the seemingly infinite numbers of variations on the theme of disease forgery (Feldman and Ford 1994).

Disease pretenders are sometimes characterized as clever or practiced in their simulations, but that is not necessarily true. Rather than deriving from the skillfulness with which the deception is plied, the reason for the delay in proving disease forgery is, in most cases, because of the medical professional's time-honored desire to believe patients. A patient's presentation of his or her medical history is at the center of all diagnostic efforts. Naturally, it is difficult to make a diagnosis while simultaneously scanning for the possibility of deception. There may be even slower recognition and confrontation of patients who are colleagues in medical or paramedical fields, even when the facts speak clearly of deception early on.

Case Vignettes

Patients who present with factitial blood disorders (anemia, bleeding) typically need medical equipment to carry out their ruses. They often work as health care professionals and thus have access to such equipment. Factitious anemia and bleeding disorders commonly involve heparin or bishydroxycoumarin, or ingestion of rat poison, which contains warfarin derivatives. Though anemia through self-induced phlebotomy has been reported many times as well, increased clotting time (i.e., slower clotting) is the usual presentation of a factitious bleeding disorder. Decreased clotting time (i.e., faster clotting) is among the few medical anomalies not yet reported in factitious disorder.

Case 2

A 28-year-old head nurse, functioning well at her job, asked for psychiatric help after being told to do so by the director of nursing. She came, she said, because of her "grim diagnosis of leukemia." After a few months of psychiatric treatment, she indicated that she had received maximal psychological help; nevertheless, she suggested continued meetings because she wanted "to learn how to help patients who are dying."

The patient was seen not only as courageous but also as an example of the ideal of the profession. She was often at work with her uniform stained from a nosebleed, yet she was noted to be careful and giving to her sick patients.

It was then discovered that she had falsely reported attendance at a nearby hospital oncology clinic. Confronted with that fact and the suspicion that her bleeding was from self-administered anticoagulants, she confessed to her psychiatrist. He asked about her motivation: "What made you do this?" She responded that many months before, a routine hematology examination revealed "some form of anemia." Though the anemia did not show up on subsequent tests, the patient indicated in a vague way that she wished to "find out for sure"; she then chose the use of heparin in order to keep herself within physicians' attention. Her mother subsequently reported that the patient had had a history of other illnesses where suspicions of a factitial etiology had been raised. As a professional, she clearly identified too closely with sick patients.

The illogical reasoning of this nurse is frequently presented in a defensive way by other factitial patients when their deceptions are uncovered. Sometimes a bit of detective work unmasks the patient, as in the following case of a factitial gastroenterologic disorder.

Case 3

A 23-year-old active-duty clerk in an Army medical unit was treated for diarrhea but was sent back to duty after the problem subsided. When it recurred and persisted, it was decided that the clerk needed a more intensive work-up at a medical center.

While in the hospital, the patient complained repeatedly about the diarrhea, which consisted of at least five or six watery or semi-solid bowel movements per day. There was no blood or mucus. Throughout and following the work-up, she was asked about, but vigorously denied, the use of cathartics.

At the end of the exhaustive work-up, the cause of the diarrhea remained a mystery. An enterprising medical resident then undertook an experiment, placing some sodium hydroxide on the patient's stool. The sample turned a startling and definitive pink, immediately establishing the diagnosis of factitious disorder. This color change, due to a chemical reaction, will occur only when a base such as sodium hydroxide comes in contact with the agent phenolphthalein; phenolphthalein is the active ingredient in many over-the-counter cathartics as well as an acid/base indicator.

When confronted, the patient again denied use of cathartics; when pressed by the assembled physicians, including the psychiatrist, she complained that she could not talk in a room full of doctors. Later, while alone with the psychiatrist, she indicated that she had suffered a genuine bout of diarrhea while on active duty; it had subsided, but she had brought it back by her secret use of phenolphthalein. She claimed her reason, like that of the nurse in Case 2, was that she wanted to "find out what really was wrong."

Another way in which patients falsify disease is through factitious dermatitis (dermatitis artefacta), which sometimes involves self-injection of foreign materials under the surface of the skin. Such patients commonly include nurses and other hospital or laboratory personnel—anyone with access to injection equipment. In these cases, diagnostic acumen, sometimes involving biopsy, is essential.

Case 4

A 48-year-old registered nurse was admitted to a hospital because of slight fever and irregularly occurring nodules in her thigh muscles and trunk. These nodules were pruritic but not tender. The odd characteristics and distribution of the lesions led to an early presumptive diagnosis of factitious disease, if not Munchausen syndrome. The patient absolutely denied any self-injection. While the patient was still hospitalized, a muscle biopsy was performed, and the content of the nodule was determined to be talc. The diagnosis was presented to the patient and her husband, both of whom were irate, denying that self-harm had ever occurred. The patient was lost to immediate follow-up but died approximately a year later at another hospital from a talc embolus.

Case 5

A 44-year-old microbiologist was in the hospital for a third repair of a skin graft to her buttocks. Despite meticulous care to the graft area, the patient developed repeated infections that threatened sloughing of the double-thickness graft.

Material from the oozing wound showed pure *Staphylococcus aureus.* The infectious disease consultant immediately became suspicious of factitious behavior. A search uncovered a small syringe (a number 16 needle) between the cushions of one of the chairs in her room. Material from this syringe contained the same pure bacterial culture, which was assumed to have been taken from bacteriology laboratory sources to which the patient had easy access. A report received subsequently from a neighboring hospital indicated that this same patient had an episode of "undulant fever" (fairly rare in New England) while the patient was hospitalized at that institution. The patient subsequently admitted to causing the undulant fever but continued to deny having tampered with her graft.

Vicarious Disease Forgery: Factitious Disorder by Proxy

By far the most sinister entry in DSM-IV for willful disease fabrication or induction is factitious disorder by proxy (FDP), considered more fully elsewhere in this book. This phenomenon is often referred to as *Munchausen syndrome by proxy, Munchausen by proxy,* or *Munchausen syndrome by proxy abuse.* Caregivers (typically mothers) produce signs and symptoms of disease in their children and then present them, with apparent great concern, for treatment (Black 1981; Meadow 1977, 1995). FDP may stem in part from a symbiotic relationship in which it is difficult for the abusive parent to recognize her own boundaries. Another conjecture is that the mother creates symptoms in her child, then cares for the child's sick body in the way she wishes for care to be rendered to her own. Some parents have been found to abuse through disease falsification many or all of their children (Alexander et al. 1990). FDP has without exaggeration been termed a *perversion of mothering* (Schreier 1992), though in a small number of cases, fathers or others are the perpetrators.

Borderline Diagnosis

Patients with factitious disorder, an Axis I diagnosis, may satisfy the criteria for other mental disorders as well. The diagnosis that seems to have the most consistent clinical congruence is borderline personality disorder (Freyberger et al. 1994; Nadelson 1979; Ries 1980), coded on Axis II. Borderline personality disorder seems particularly to apply to the group of factitious disorder patients who work in medical settings (Nadelson 1979). The borderline personality is marked by unstable interpersonal relationships as well as rage, impulsivity, self-mutilation and/or suicide attempts, and rapid shifts of mood. The borderline patient alternately idealizes and intensely denigrates other people, and the patient's own goals and values are similarly uncertain and changeable (American Psychiatric Association 1994).

For the patient with factitious disorder and borderline personality, disease falsification provides a focus for anger and transiently stabilizes a continually shifting affective state. In some cases, borderline patients' experiences with illness and death during their formative years have helped direct them toward the subsequent medical dissimulations (Chapman 1957; Cramer et al. 1971). In addition, many studies have reported a strong correlation between a history of physical and/or sexual abuse and the development of borderline personality disorder (Gunderson and Sabo 1993; Gunderson and Zanarini 1989; Herman and van der Kolk 1987; Herman et al. 1989; Paris and Zweig-Frank 1992; Stone 1990; Terr 1991; Westen et al. 1990; van der Kolk et al. 1991). Though there is no confirming evidence at present, it is possible that many factitious disorder patients, especially those with borderline character pathology, were abused as children. For such individuals, the psychic trauma contributing to the borderline personality structure may also contribute to a tendency to chronic disease simulation. Clearly, disease mimicry can be a mode of interaction in which a powerful figure (a physician) is controlled in a manner that expresses an ambivalence between the inherent dependency of all children and the hostile resentment of children who have been abused. The factitious behavior thus gratifies the borderline patient because it temporarily stabilizes painful affective shifts by substituting the physician as the target in the place of the self.

A Sickness Spectrum

A spectrum of sickness is presented in Table 1–1, which places "false patients" (the factitious disorder and malingering groups) at one end (Category C) and "real patients" at the other end (Category A). A wholly "real" patient, it is noted here again, is an "ideal" rather than a frequent reality.

Real Patients

Real patients are viewed as authentic because they have fallen ill only through accident or chance, rather than because their emotional needs have found expression in somatic complaints. They are assumed not to have acted as agents of causation of their illnesses, even unconsciously. Though stress from the environment may in some cases have impaired their immune mechanisms, increasing their susceptibility to illness, this same feature could occur in most people, and they are still "victims." The illnesses of real patients are located and contained within the space of their bodies, bounded by their skin. The stressor, or etiology for sickness, is that which is usually defined for purely physical illness (e.g., toxin, infectious agent, trauma, or cancer).

The status of the real patient is honorable and socially respected, and the seeking of the position it confers is understandable. (Consider the change in the social perception of a man who is drunk and is therefore avoided or "invisible"; when he becomes a patient in response to bleeding varices, he is instantly given attention, addressed courteously by name, and given a clean bed and food.) Further, the real patient cooperates in order to shed patienthood as soon as possible (Parsons 1951).

Somatoform Disorders and Abnormal Illness Behavior

Humans share some wish for caretaking, and patients with genuine ailments may, at times, magnify symptoms in a search for nurturance. As noted at the beginning of this chapter, nonpsychiatric clinicians generally polarize the universe of patients into the real versus the false. Within this type of clinical thinking, the group with physical complaints that coexist with psychiatric diagnoses are relegated to some murky point not quite in either domain.

In fact, between the idealized real patient and the wholly false patient are those with somatoform disorders. The group of patients placed in this portion of the spectrum includes, according to DSM-IV nomenclature: somatization disorder (the patient offers polysymptomatic complaints over many years); conversion disorder (the patient experiences symptoms or deficits affecting voluntary motor or sensory function); undifferentiated somatoform disorder (the patient reports unexplained physical complaints that do not reach the level of the criteria for somatization disorder); pain disorder (severe pain is the prominent focus with psychological factors judged to be significant); hypochondriasis (the patient is preoccupied with the fear of serious disease, causing impairment of functioning); body dysmorphic disorder (an intense preoccupation with a mild or imagined defect in appearance); and somatoform disorder not otherwise specified (a residual category for phenomena such as pseudocyesis, the false belief of being pregnant).

Patients with somatoform disorders present with symptoms that suggest a general medical condition but which are not fully supported by objective medical data. Such patients are grouped within Category B in Table 1–1.

Early psychoanalytic ideas on the etiology of somatic fixation were focused on the presumed significance of childhood experience. Psychoanalytic models of mind-body relationships presented some disease states as symbolic or metaphoric encapsulations of conflict. For example, a peptic ulcer crater was once viewed as an "internal bite," a physical representation of the conflict in the oral stage of development. There is less emphasis now among psychiatrists on the exclusive use of symbol or conflict translated into somatic manifestation. Peptic ulcer is currently viewed, for example, as causally related, in most cases, to infection with the bacterium *Helicobacter pylori* (Soll 1996).

Patients with somatoform disorders are strongly influenced by psychological factors, and most nonpsychiatric physicians will not accord them the honor allotted to individuals in Category A. Even without attempting consciously to deceive, such patients are viewed as if they were "sailing under false colors," presenting themselves to physicians as if they had real disease. The terms abnormal illness behavior (Pilowsky 1969) and somatic amplifiers (Barsky 1992) have been used in attempts at categorization of such individuals without imposing the absolutely pejorative connotation of "crock." Nevertheless, their psychiatric diagnoses bring somatoform disorder patients into the medical structure because psychiatrists are physicians. Though lacking real disease (and/or a biomedical etiology), somatoform patients are legitimate patients.

Another group of patients often considered suspect as to the authenticity of their physical complaints consists of those with work-related injuries. Some may indeed have a compensation neurosis (Ellard 1974; Rickarby 1979) motivated by intra- and interpersonal psychological needs (e.g., a need for victimization, for nurturance, or for some type of intangible reward). Such patients also may be motivated to obtain financial compensation, a factor that contributes significantly to health care costs worldwide. To illustrate, continual use of computer keyboards caused an Australian epidemic in the early 1980s of what was termed repetitive strain injury (RSI). A subset of workers complaining of such injuries presented overtly magnified or even spurious wrist symptoms ascribable to work, earning the designation goldenpaw (Auerbach 1984); these individuals would be viewed within DSM-IV as malingerers. However, it was also noted that the majority of afflicted workers were not attempting to perpetrate fraud (Miller and Topliss 1988). Rather, the mild to moderate discomfort of continual keyboard use was exacerbated in the minds of the workers by the changing social climate of an industrialized nation in which welfare had become increasingly salient and work-related physical ailments increasingly socially acceptable. In essence, the diagnosis of RSI was seen as self-generating; once made, the RSI diagnosis was continually reinforced by well-meaning public agencies. The epidemic finally abated after clinicians pointed to the importance, and the cost, of such social factors (Ireland 1992). Many patients disabled by work-related injuries of little objective consequence are people who have worked hard, often beginning at a very early age, and who also have difficulty acknowledging their own dependency needs. Some yearn for care for themselves but feel forced to care for others. A patient who eagerly sought hospitalization for a minor ailment expressed the contradictory pull in one breath: "I can't keep working . . . I have to."

Malingering

The distinction between malingering, which is not a DSM-IV diagnosis, and factitious disorder, which is a DSM-IV diagnosis, can be subtle. As a result, the terms unfortunately are often used interchangeably by clinicians. The malingerer wants to avoid work, evade or escape from a distasteful environment or situation (military service or criminal prosecution), obtain money (from lawsuits, disability or insurance claims, or other sources of compensation), and/or appropriate other external gains (opioid medications). Thus, the symptom production or exaggeration in malingering is prompted by a specific external incentive (e.g., Binder and Rohling 1996); in contrast, the goal driving the symptom production in factitious disorders, including Munchausen syndrome, is the "sick role" itself.

Case 6

A man was brought to a general hospital from prison. In the midst of feeling depressed he had, he said, swallowed razor blades. A radiologic exam in prison clearly showed two razor blades in his duodenum. After laparotomy recovered two blades (carefully wrapped in tape), the inmate confessed that he wanted some time out of prison. Although he lost "good time" by carrying out the ruse (his hospital stay did not count toward his prison sentence), he said it was worth it. It was a vacation without pay, but still a vacation.

Convicts frequently seek surcease from dismal prison life by this route. Many inmates say that the worst enemy in that extremely hostile environment is boredom. Some have learned that razor blades wrapped in radiolucent tape and swallowed are not, in themselves, a risk to life but still appear on X ray as sharp steel, often mandating surgery and hospital time.

Individuals who malinger may do so occasionally or chronically. As indicated, some environments—such as military, prison, and legal settings—are associated with an increased incidence of malingering. Malingerers who pursue contrived malpractice suits and insurance claims may find sympathetic juries, as well as lawyers eager to advocate on the litigants' behalf.

In a sense, malingerers may have, as a group, a chronic grievance. Some feel strongly that advantage has been taken of them and that they need to right a wrong. Others are more sociopathic, with histories of other forms of illegal deception or even outright theft; through their malingering, they simply wish to steal what they cannot obtain in another way and present no moral excuse for such behavior.

A number of authors maintain that such patients need, and perhaps deserve, psychiatric help, and that they have been forced into a category that socially condemns them. In contrast, this writer believes that such behavior is outside of allowable medical limits. Once malingered illness has been detected, consequent physical damage should be repaired but the patient should not be treated psychiatrically for the malingering itself.

Most of the literature on the subject of malingering is aimed at ways to detect the malingerer. Tests such as Minnesota Multiphasic Personality Inventory may be used to uncover those feigning psychosis. Restricting the gratification the malingerer obtains from his or her sickness may work as well, both as a diagnostic maneuver and as a deterrent. For example, professional ruses, such as frightening the suspected malingerer with an ostentatious display of large needles "required" for diagnosis, can lead to confession (although even real patients may be dissuaded from medical care under such circumstances).

However, malingerers are generally found to maintain their symptoms until some settlement or restitution is made. The problems encountered clinically are usually complex.

Case 7

A 64-year-old man, injured in an accident at work, had consultations with a series of surgeons, internists, and neurologists before finally seeing a psychiatrist. His initial injury at age 34 had led to a below-knee amputation. Subsequent revisions of the stump continued off and on through a large portion of his adult life. Because of pain, he was given morphine over a long period of time, resulting in addiction. The patient was viewed early in the course of treatment as someone who magnified symptoms. Worker's Compensation paid for his medications, physicians, and hospitalization over the years. He continued to pursue with great intensity the possibility of an additional sum above his monthly disability payment.

This abbreviated vignette contains elements of the problems usually encountered in chronic injury. Malingering was discussed at several points as a likely etiology for this man's ongoing problems. He spent much of his time in bed. Some of his physicians felt that he avoided rehabilitation and had no motivation toward better functioning. He was active in a veterans' organization and often implied falsely that his disability was a result of military combat.

The practitioner encounters a real challenge in attempting to distinguish the patient's motivation for concrete personal gain from the omnipresent potential of an authentic physical cause for complaint, and this challenge is depicted in Case 7. Is the patient more a malingerer than a sufferer?

The motivation for tangible external gain is, in reality, often interwoven with a wish for care, support, or a better sense of self. Thus, both the sick role and the potential for compensation or other gain appeal to the individual. For example, from an intrapsychic standpoint, a cash settlement is also an acknowledgment of the patient's innocence and right to an aggrieved status. In this way, false patients in both the factitious disorder and malingering categories overlap at times. In Chapter 5, the authors discuss these issues in greater detail.

Conclusion

Psychiatry, as medicine, science, and social force, has marginally dispelled the fog of moral condemnation surrounding some human failings. Dynamic explanations have tended to lift the stigma from behaviors by substituting psychic mechanisms for moral judgments. Thus, one direction of psychiatric nosology is toward establishment of a kinder view of human diversity. So-called biologic psychiatry has had a similar social effect far beyond diagnostic and therapeutic intent; explanations for behavior, affect, and thought focused on brain function push the conceptual burden of personal failure away from the responsibility or "choice" of the individual. As explanatory mechanisms for self-damaging behaviors evolve, it is hoped that they too will decrease stigma; at the same time, they should not simultaneously erase individual responsibility to society and law.

Although therapy with malingerers has been suggested, and positive therapeutic results for patients with full-blown Munchausen syndrome have been reported (Mayo and Haggerty 1984), the view expressed here is that we do better to impose social and legal restraints rather than embark upon psychiatric treatment. The psychiatric consultant is well advised not to begin a psychotherapeutic relationship with a patient suspected by the referring physician of disease simulation. Too often, this referral is a prelude to "splitting": the patient's pitting one doctor against another. The diagnosis of Munchausen syndrome is usually made by the referring professional, and the psychiatrist can better help the clinical situation by finding a way quickly to end the clinical episode. Legal recourse is possible when malingering occurs, and certainly a charge of child abuse should be pursued when there is strong evidence of FDP. Those who mimic disease need to prove their interest in treatment if they request it. The therapist should reserve judgment about the sincerity of the motivation until time proves otherwise. However, we should know that we still can define that which we cannot reliably cure.

The public's increasing fascination with false illness is reflected in recent talk-radio and television "infotainment" programs. The families of such patients, however, may be more perplexed and hurt than fascinated. Of course, health care systems are burdened as well. Education may help the general public, family members, and health care professionals achieve perspective. A readable book on disease forgery designed for both health care providers and the public has appeared (Feldman and Ford 1994).

References

Aduan RP, Fauci AS, Dale DC, et al: Factitious fever and self-induced infection: a report of 32 cases and review of the literature. Ann Intern Med 90:230–242, 1979

Alexander R, Smith W, Stevenson R: Serial Munchausen by proxy. Pediatrics 86:581–585, 1990

American Psychiatric Association: Diagnostic and Statistical Manual of Mental Disorders, Fourth Edition. Washington, DC, American Psychiatric Association, 1994

Asher R: Munchausen's syndrome. Lancet 1:339–341, 1951

Auerbach M: RSI or kangaroo paw. Med J Aust 142:237, 1984

Baile WF Jr, Kuehn CV, Straker D: Factitious cancer. Psychosomatics 33:100–104, 1992

Barsky A: Amplification, somatization, and the somatoform disorders. Psychosomatics 33:28–34, 1992

Binder LM, Rohling ML: Money matters: a meta-analytic review of the effects of financial incentives on recovery after closed-head injury. Am J Psychiatry 153:7–10, 1996

Black D: The extended Munchausen syndrome. Br J Psychiatry 138:466–469, 1981

Chapman JS: Peregrinating problem patients: Munchausen's syndrome. JAMA 165:927–933, 1957

Clark E, Melnick S: The Munchausen syndrome or problem of hospital hobos. Am J Med 25:6–12, 1958

Cramer B, Gershberg MR, Stern M: Munchausen syndrome: its relationship to malingering, hysteria and the physician-patient relationship. Arch Gen Psychiatry 24:573–78, 1971

Ellard J: Psychological reactions to compensable injury. Med J Aust 2:349–355, 1974

Feldman MD, Ford CV: Patient or Pretender: Inside the Strange World of Factitious Disorders. New York, Wiley, 1994

Folks DG, Kinney FC: The role of psychological factors in dermatologic conditions. Psychosomatics 33:45–54, 1992

Ford CV: The Somatizing Disorders: Illness as a Way of Life. New York, Elsevier, 1983

Freyberger H, Nordmeyer JP, Freyberger H, et al: Patients suffering from factitious disorders in the clinico-psychosomatic consultation liaison service: psychodynamic processes, psychotherapeutic initial care and clinicointerdisciplinary cooperation. Psychother Psychosom 62:108–122, 1994

Gunderson JG, Sabo AN: The phenomenological and conceptual interface between borderline personality disorder and PTSD. Am J Psychiatry 150:19–28, 1993

Gunderson JG, Zanarini MC: Pathogenesis of borderline personality disorder, in American Psychiatric Press Review of Psychiatry, Vol 8. Edited by Tasman A, Hales RE, Frances AJ. Washington, DC, American Psychiatric Press, 1989, pp 25–48

Herman J, van der Kolk BA: Traumatic antecedents of borderline personality disorder, in Psychological Trauma. Edited by van der Kolk BA. Washington, DC, American Psychiatric Press, 1987, pp 111–126

Herman JL, Perry JC, van der Kolk BA: Childhood trauma in borderline personality disorder. Am J Psychiatry 146:490–495, 1989

Hoeper E, Nycz G, Regier D, et al: Diagnosis of mental disorder in adults and increased use of health services in four outpatient settings. Am J Psychiatry 137:207–210, 1980

Ireland DC: The Australian experience with cumulative trauma disorders, in Occupational Disorders of the Upper Extremity. Edited by Millender LC, Louis DS, Simmons BP. New York, Churchill Livingstone, 1992, pp 79–88

Lipsitt D: Medical and psychological management of "crocks." Psychiatr Med 1:15–25, 1970

Luce JM: The legacy of Baron Munchausen. Pharos 41:19–23, 1978

Mayo J, Haggerty J: Long term psychotherapy of Munchausen syndrome. Am J Psychother 38:571–579, 1984

Meadow R: What is, and what is not, "Munchausen syndrome by proxy?" Arch Dis Child 72:534–538, 1995

Meadow R: Munchausen syndrome by proxy: the hinterland of child abuse. Lancet 1:343–345, 1977

Miller MH, Topliss DJ: Chronic upper limb pain syndrome. Repetitive strain injury in the Australian workforce: a systematic cross sectional rheumatological study of 229 patients. J Rheumatol 15:1705–1712, 1988

Nadelson T: The Munchausen spectrum: borderline character features. Gen Hosp Psychiatry 1:11–17, 1979

Nadelson T: Psychological factors in upper extremity disorders: pain as a paradigm, in Occupational Disorders of the Upper Extremity. Edited by Millender LC, Louis DS, Simmons BP. New York, Churchill Livingstone, 1992, pp 215–226

Paris J, Zweig-Frank H: A critical review of the role of childhood sexual abuse in the etiology of borderline personality disorder. Can J Psychiatry 37:125–128, 1992

Parsons T: The Social System. New York, Free Press, 1951

Pilowsky I: Abnormal illness behavior. Br J Med Psychol 42:347–351, 1969

Reich P, Gottfried LA: Factitious disorders in a teaching hospital. Ann Intern Med 99:240–247, 1983

Rickarby G: Compensation neurosis and the psycho-social requirements of the family. Br J Med Psychol 52:333–335, 1979

Ries R: DSM-III differential diagnosis of Munchausen's syndrome. J Nerv Ment Dis 168:629–631, 1980

Schreier HA: The perversion of mothering: Munchausen syndrome by proxy. Bull Menninger Clin 56:421–436, 1992

Soll AH: Medical treatment of peptic ulcer disease. JAMA 275:622–629, 1996

Stone MH: Abuse and abusiveness in borderline personality disorder, in Family Environment and Borderline Personality Disorder. Edited by Links P. Washington, DC, American Psychiatric Press, 1990, pp 131–148

Terr LC: Childhood traumas: an outline and overview. Am J Psychiatry 148:10–203, 1991

van der Kolk BA, Perry JC, Herman JL: Childhood origins of self-destructive behavior. Am J Psychiatry 148:1665–1671, 1991

Voiss DV: Occupational injury. Fact, fantasy, or fraud? Neurol Clin 13:431–446, 1995

Westen D, Ludolph P, Misle B, et al: Physical and sexual abuse in adolescent girls with borderline personality disorder. Am J Orthopsychiatry 60:55–66, 1990

CHAPTER 2

Current Overview of Factitious Physical Disorders

Stuart J. Eisendrath, M.D.

Factitious physical disorders refer to those conditions that individuals willfully create by producing signs and/or symptoms of physical illness. Although Asher (1951) drew attention to these disorders with his paper "Munchausen's Syndrome," they had already been identified centuries earlier (Gavin 1838). Even today, nearly everyone is aware of his or her own amplification of physical symptoms at certain times to fulfill some psychological need. For example, a young child who experiences the entry of a new sibling into the family may elaborate somatic symptoms as a means of refocusing parental attention. Thus, factitious behaviors can be conceptualized as representing a spectrum that ranges from normal adaptive functioning to severe disability. Factitious behaviors are typically considered to become a disorder only when they significantly or persistently interfere with normal functioning (Folks 1995).

Asher, however, focused physician awareness on the most severe form of factitious disorders, Munchausen syndrome, with his 1951 article in *The Lancet*. European children had heard the tales of Baron Münchhausen who, in essence, was the equivalent of the American folklore hero Paul Bunyan (Nickl 1992). As described in Chapter 1, Asher selected the Baron's name for this syndrome because these patients often told fantastic tales of their wanderings, life adventures, and medical experiences.

The term *Munchausen* has been so exotically appealing that

many physicians have failed to recognize that most patients with factitious disorders do not suffer from the syndrome. Reich and Gottfried (1983) estimated that only 10% of patients with factitious disorders have Munchausen syndrome. These patients have an essentially intractable course of illnesses and hospitalizations. In addition, patients with Munchausen syndrome not only produce signs or symptoms of disease but also wander widely, have sociopathic features, give astounding medical histories, and have a life filled with little else besides their illnesses. These patients are generally regarded as refractory to psychiatric intervention. Most patients with factitious physical disorder, in contrast, have intermittent episodes of illness, do not wander, and have stable social systems. They often have families and may hold responsible jobs, frequently in the nursing profession. Thus, most patients with factitious physical disorder are more amenable to treatment interventions than the subset of patients with Munchausen syndrome.

Epidemiology

The epidemiology of factitious physical disorders is based upon data that are limited. Many cases go unidentified by physicians. Other cases may be reported in the medical literature multiple times and by different authors (Duffy 1992; Ifudu et al. 1992). Even when factitious physical disorders are identified, factors such as insurance reimbursement and litigation concerns may influence whether the diagnosis is recorded as such in the medical record. Nonetheless, various authors have reached some agreement (Folks and Houck 1993; Taylor and Hyler 1993). It appears that approximately two-thirds of patients with Munchausen syndrome are male. In the more common non-Munchausen forms of factitious physical disorders, females outnumber males by a 3:1 ratio (Freyberger et al. 1994). It is possible that the predominance of males with Munchausen syndrome is related to the acculturation directing poorly adapting males toward more overt sociopathy. The non-Munchausen patients appear to share features with patients having somatoform diagnoses such as somatization disorder, who express conflicts without overt acting out.

The best epidemiologic studies relate to specific illnesses

evaluated under careful conditions. One study of fever of unknown origin carried out at the National Institutes of Health found that 6.5% of 200 cases were factitious (Herzberg and Wolff 1972). In a study at the National Institute for Allergy and Infectious Disease, Aduan et al. (1979) reported that the fevers of 9.3% of their 343 patients were factitious. Another study of the same condition at Stanford University revealed that 2.2% of 506 cases were factitious (Rumans and Vosti 1978). More recently, Knockaert and colleagues (1992) found that 3.5% of 199 cases were factitious, a rate higher than that associated with drug-related fevers (3.0%). In an interesting study of urinary calculi, Gault and colleagues (1988) discovered that 3.5% of stones were factitious in origin; they were primarily quartz, feldspar, and other exogenous minerals. These studies suggest that factitious disorders play a significant role in health care utilization.

Factitious physical disorders usually develop during the third or fourth decade of life. There are often precursors to the behavior during childhood and adolescence. Histories obtained from these individuals commonly include an unexpectedly large number of childhood illnesses and operations. Some of these histories feature a childhood record of telling lies frequently and easily; in some instances, the lies involve alleged sexual abuse that is later disproved (Barker and Howell 1994; Rand 1993).

A variety of psychiatric diagnoses have been associated with factitious physical disorders. Nadelson (1979) suggests that many of these patients suffer from borderline personality disorder. This type of individual may create marked splitting of medical ward staffs. Staff members who have been seen as "good" by the patient are often extremely sympathetic; staff seen as "bad" may be drawn into marked conflict with the patient. When the factitious diagnosis is finally made, the staff may be similarly split into sympathetic and angry camps.

Other authors have noted a broader spectrum of comorbid psychiatric diagnoses. Earle and Folks (1986) identified depression as a major component in a case that was amenable to pharmacologic intervention. It appears likely that when depression is present as a comorbid disorder, this feature actually bodes well for treatment. The effective treatments available for depression can decrease the affective state that may be driving much of the factitious behavior.

Most clinicians concur that overt psychosis is rare in factitious patients with physical disorders. Nonetheless, Spivak and colleagues (1994) have hypothesized that an underlying psychosis may be present in some of these patients and that the factitious physical disorder actually helps the individual avoid personality fragmentation. It does so by helping to organize the patient's relationships with the world into the familiar and well-controlled framework of the medical setting. During treatment of patients with factitious disorders, some patients with the tendency for personality disorganization have benefited from judicious use of neuroleptic medications on a time-limited basis (Fras and Coughlin 1971).

Clinical Features

Any individual studying factitious physical disorders soon appreciates human creativity. Almost every illness known to humankind has been produced factitiously. For example, factitious fevers have been produced by holding a thermometer near a light bulb, drinking a hot liquid before a temperature is taken, or injecting a bacterial culture intravenously. One individual simulated fevers by rapidly contracting and relaxing the anal sphincter in order to produce friction heat, thereby elevating rectal thermometer readings (Aduan et al. 1979); some have induced actual fever with pyrogenic medications (Nordmeyer 1994). Others have chosen to induce different signs and symptoms by injecting egg protein into the urethra to simulate proteinuria, injecting insulin to mimic the hypoglycemia of an insulinoma, or taking diuretics to produce the appearance of familial hypokalemia.

Laboratory abnormalities of many types have been produced factitiously (e.g., anemia, hematuria, hyperamylasuria, and profound coagulopathies). Wallach (1994) has cataloged the multitude of abnormalities produced factitiously (Table 2–1).

Conditions as diverse as systemic lupus erythematosus (Apfelbaum and Williams 1994), chronic diarrhea (Topazian and Binder 1994), pheochromocytoma (Kailasam et al. 1995; Keiser 1991), pancytopenia (Ford et al. 1984), Goodpasture's syndrome (Ifudu et al. 1992), Cushing's syndrome (Anderson et al. 1993), AIDS (Bialer and Wallack 1990), and glossopharyngeal neuralgia (Scully et al. 1995) have been factitiously created by resourceful patients. Individuals have been remarkably inventive. One patient cajoled a physician to supply him with testosterone injections. He next convinced another physician to provide corticosteroids and thyroid hormone. Finally, he persuaded a third physician that he had panhypopituitarism that required long-term treatment with these multiple hormones.

Table 2–1. Examples of factitious disorders in which the laboratory has a role

Manifestation or disorder simulated	Cause
Hypoglycemia	Administration of insulin
Hyperthyroidism	Ingestion of liothyronine or thyroxine
Pheochromocytoma	Self-injection of metaraminol or epinephrine
Hypokalemia	Laxative abuse, induced vomiting, diuretic abuse
Bleeding diathesis	Sodium warfarin ingestion
Anemia	Self-administered phlebotomy
Hemoptysis	Addition of blood, self-induced trauma
AIDS	Fictitious history
Mydriasis	Self-administered homatropine eye drops
Diarrhea	Excess ingestion of phenolphthalein or castor oil
Vomiting	Ipecac abuse
Urinary calculi	Materials added to urine, stones inserted into urethra
Goodpasture's syndrome	Adding blood to urine, false history
Hematuria	Contamination with external blood or meat; sodium warfarin ingestion; addition of povidone-iodine to urine, causing false-positive dipstick result
Bacteriuria	Urine contamination in vivo or in vitro

Source. Adapted from Wallach 1994.

DSM-IV (American Psychiatric Association 1994) has described the criteria for factitious physical disorders (Table 2–2). These criteria include the intentional production or feigning of physical disorders in order to assume the sick role. There is no obvious external gain associated with the deceptive behavior.

Deceptions can occur at three levels (Eisendrath 1984). Some patients give a fictitious history alone in order to convince unwary physicians of their illness. Acquired immunodeficiency syndrome and cancer diagnoses have been made by some physi-

Table 2–2. DSM-IV criteria for factitious disorder

A. Intentional production or feigning of physical or psychological signs or symptoms

B. The motivation for the behavior is to assume the sick role

C. External incentives for the behavior (such as economic gain, avoiding legal responsibility, or improving physical well-being, as in malingering) are absent

Code based on type:

300.16 With predominantly psychological signs and symptoms: if psychological signs and symptoms predominate in the clinical presentation

300.19 With predominantly physical signs and symptoms: if physical signs and symptoms predominate in the clinical presentation

300.19 With combined psychological and physical signs and symptoms: if both psychological and physical signs and symptoms are present but neither predominates in the clinical presentation

300.19 Factitious disorder not otherwise specified
This category includes disorders with factitious symptoms that do not meet criteria for a specific factitious disorder. An example is factitious disorder by proxy: the intentional production or feigning of physical or psychological signs or symptoms in another person who is under the individual's care for the purpose of indirectly assuming the sick role

Source. Reprinted with permission from American Psychiatric Association: Diagnostic and Statistical Manual of Mental Disorders, 4th Editon. Washington, DC, American Psychiatric Association, 1994, pp. 474–475. Copyright 1994 American Psychiatric Association.

cians who tacitly accepted the history provided by a new patient (Churchill et al. 1994; Feldman and Escalona 1991; Songer 1995). Another group of patients has simulated medical illness. These patients have performed acts such as adding blood to urine to simulate hematuria or elevating thermometer readings artificially by applying heat. The third category of deception includes those patients who actually create a pathophysiological state. These individuals may do things such as inject themselves with bacteria to produce sepsis or take thyroid hormone to create hyperthyroid states.

Typically, individuals with factitious disorders have some association with the health care field (Aduan et al. 1979; Cramer et al. 1971). They commonly work in a health-related occupation, or someone in their family is a health care employee (Freyberger et al. 1994). They may create an episode of factitious illness when faced with a life stressor such as a loss (Geracioti et al. 1987). For example, a well-functioning clinical nurse developed hypoglycemic episodes shortly after losing a highly desired pregnancy to miscarriage. The hypoglycemia was eventually diagnosed with C-peptide studies as due to exogenous insulin administration, and she entered psychotherapy. In another case, the head nurse of a critical care unit developed abdominal abscesses during periods of marital discord. A house officer discovered her injecting a fecal specimen into her abdominal wall during one hospitalization. She eventually revealed having injected herself several times previously. These two cases illustrate that many patients with factitious physical disorders have stable work histories. They also may have strong family connections, even if dysfunctional, that provide settings for psychiatric interventions that are far superior to those possible with the ever-shifting Munchausen syndrome patients.

As noted, individuals with Munchausen syndrome are significantly different from the majority of patients with factitious physical disorder; they are itinerant hospital seekers, usually covering a number of cities and states in their travels. In the past, this feature led to designations such as "peregrinating problem patients" or "hospital hoboes." These individuals do often tell fantastic tales that have been labeled as pseudologia fantastica by some authors (Cramer et al. 1971; Ford 1996). The stories often include an element of impostorship where the individual portrays him- or herself in some grandiose role, such as a war hero. Usually, however, these individuals give clues to the listener of their impostorship because, to feel satisfied, they need to demonstrate how cleverly they have duped their caregivers. Although seen in a number of personality disorders and not confined to factitious disorder patients, the pseudologia fantastica that patients with Munchausen syndrome use can been considered an attempt at wish fulfillment and regulation of self-esteem (Ford et al. 1988). For an individual with little realistic accomplishment, pseudologia fantastica may be an attempt, albeit an illusory one, to enhance one's self-concept.

Diagnosis

Factitious disorders often exist for a lengthy period before they are correctly diagnosed. Reich and Gottfried (1983) estimated that the average factitious cellulitis required 6 years to be identified. The delay in diagnosis is unfortunate because it often leads to inappropriate interventions and iatrogenic complications. Additionally, the interval before the factitious etiology is discovered may lead to enormous financial drains on the health care system. A British report described one individual who was called the "Million Dollar Man" because of expenses deriving from his factitious physical disorder (Powell and Boast 1993). A patient at a San Francisco medical center generated charges of over 1 million dollars in a 1-year period because of factitiously produced aplastic anemia (Eisendrath, unpublished observations). The patient had induced complete bone marrow suppression by the use of the chemotherapy agent busulfan and required extensive transfusion support. Clearly, it is in everyone's interest to identify and appropriately treat factitious physical disorder patients as quickly as possible (Cohen et al. 1985).

A number of clues exist that may help the clinician identify factitious disorders. One common finding is that the medical condition does not respond to seemingly correct medical treatment. Examples include wounds or abscesses that do not heal despite appropriate skin grafting or antibiotic treatment. As noted previously, another important clue is the occupational history of the individual. Nurses, medical technicians, paramedics, and other health care workers appear most prone to develop factitious physical disorders. These individuals may oscillate between being caregivers and care-receivers as they vacillate in their psychological conflicts.

Another clue is the sheer amount of medical care these patients may have consumed. Despite their relatively young age, these patients have usually had a remarkably large number of medical interventions. Indeed, the eagerness to undergo invasive diagnostic and therapeutic interventions is another sign of a factitious disorder diagnosis. An additional sign that the disorder is factitious appears when the patient is notably accurate in forecasting the waxing and waning of the signs and symptoms of his or her illness. For example, one licensed practical nurse was able to predict the location and development of an abdominal abscess well in advance of any physical findings, laboratory abnormalities, or positive gallium scans. Once the factitious diagnosis was established, her prognostic powers were better understood.

Other clues to diagnosis may be revealed in observing the patient's family and friends within the hospital setting. Some of these patients will have serious medical problems that would generate concern in most families; yet, the factitious physical disorder patient is often isolated and has few visitors. This finding is especially common in the Munchausen syndrome variant, where relatives and friends have been alienated. Given a potential case of factitious physical disorder, it is wise for the physician to seek collateral sources of information. Prior physicians and hospitals, as well as any family members willing to cooperate, can provide critical information that the patient has withheld.

Differential Diagnosis

The most important diagnosis to rule out when faced with a probable factitious disorder case is a genuine medical condition that might be producing the illness (Feldman and Ford 1994). Typically, the physician can readily rule out abnormalities such as an immune dysfunction that interferes with wound healing. Once genuine disease has been excluded, the physician must consider willfully self-destructive acts such as suicide attempts or self-mutilation. Individuals committing these acts may need medical care but only as a secondary event. Also, these patients usually acknowledge their roles in creating the injuries.

In order to sharpen the factitious diagnosis, the physician must consider a number of other behaviors. Pilowsky (1978) coined the term *abnormal illness-affirming behavior* to describe the condition in which an individual amplifies signs or symptoms of illness out of proportion to the biomedical disease present. These conditions include malingering, conversion disorder, hypochondriasis, somatization disorder, and pain associated with psychological factors (formerly somatoform pain disorder). Table 2–3 shows the characteristics of and the relationships among these conditions.

Malingering and factitious disorders share the feature of conscious production of signs and symptoms (see also Chapter 1). The motivation in malingering, however, is primarily conscious and easily inferred by an outside observer. Typically, the malingerer is producing signs or symptoms in order to achieve an external gain such as monetary rewards, narcotics, or relief from a noxious situation. Patients with factitious disorders generally are aware of their role in producing their illness but do not clearly understand why they are doing so. An outside observer would have to hypothesize about the patient's unconscious mental processes to understand the motivation. Further differentiation of malingering and factitious physical disorders is discussed in Chapter 5, "Factitious Disorders and Litigation."

Differentiating whether a particular behavior is being produced consciously or unconsciously may be difficult. Overholser

Table 2–3. Abnormal illness-affirming behaviors

	Signs and symptoms	
	Production	**Motivation**
Malingering	Conscious	Conscious
Factitious disorder	Conscious	Unconscious
Conversion disorder	Unconscious	Unconscious
Somatization disorder	Unconscious	Unconscious
Hypochondriasis	Unconscious	Unconscious
Pain associated with psychological factors	Unconscious	Unconscious

Source. Adapted from Eisendrath 1984.

(1990) noted that the following factors may aid in identifying the conscious (voluntary) production of signs or symptoms: 1) direct patient admission of fabrication; 2) observation of fabrication; 3) signs or symptoms that contradict laboratory testing; 4) nonphysiologic response to treatment; and 5) physical evidence such as the finding of pills or syringes. Others consider behavior to be consciously produced when the individual must make decisions regarding timing and concealment that require judgment and intellectual activity (Teasell and Shapiro 1994). For example, if a patient was able to use a supposedly paralyzed limb when the patient felt he or she was not being watched, an observer would have to deduce a voluntary component to the paralysis.

Conversion disorder, hypochondriasis, somatization disorder, and pain associated with psychological factors all have unconscious motivations and unconscious production of signs or symptoms. These patients are unaware of their own roles in producing their disorders (Eisendrath 1995b).

Etiology

There are several ways of conceptualizing the "reasons" for factitious physical disorders. The first involves the psychodynamic functions that the behavior may serve in the individual's life (Ford 1973, 1982). One psychodynamic factor is the individual's sense of control and mastery that is achieved via the factitious behavior. Many of these patients suffered traumatic illnesses as children; the factitious disorder may allow them to feel in control as they never did in childhood. This feature is often evident in the patient who appears more calm in the face of a medical crisis than do his or her physicians.

Another prominent factor in the psychology of the factitious disorder patient is masochism. These individuals often feel marked guilt in response to feelings such as anger or sexual excitation. As a result, they may produce the factitious behavior as a means of atonement and self-punishment (Stone 1977). In some instances, the factitious disorders are based on childhood experiences of physical or sexual abuse. The disorder may become a vehicle by which the abuse is reenacted. The physician unwittingly becomes a symbolic representation of the abusing parent

(Eisendrath 1995a). The patient with factitious physical disorder may feel gratification and control in this reenactment.

In a related psychodynamic theme, the patient with factitious physical disorder may also use the illness to ventilate rage at symbolic caregivers. The rage is often the result of deprivation and mistreatment as a child. Outwitting physicians initially, the patient typically allows the deception to be detected. In this manner, the patient may feel a sense of conquest and superiority. Simultaneously, the discovery generates anger in the caregiver that reenacts earlier relationships. The patient's perception of an angry, depriving parental surrogate (the duped physician) is validation of his or her life view.

In some instances, as suggested earlier, the factitious physical disorder may represent the individual's attempt to defend against a loss. For example, if the individual suffers the death of a loved one, the activation of a factitious physical disorder may help the patient avoid focusing on the loss. The factitious disorder may also produce a substitute for the lost object by establishing a connection between the patient and a nurturing caregiver.

In contrast to the previous psychodynamic formulations, one could speculate that behavioral conditioning concepts play a key role in the onset and recurrence of the condition. As described, factitious physical disorders often have precursors in childhood. These precursors, such as a child's feigning illness for parental attention, may lead to positive reinforcement of the behaviors. Pathological amplification of the factitious behavior might occur based upon learning concepts. The individual is rewarded for sick role behavior by getting his or her needs met. This pattern of reinforcement may lay the groundwork for the later dysfunctional utilization of factitious behavior, although most children obviously do not develop full-blown factitious disorders later in life.

A factitious disorder, at least in the early stages, frequently brings the individual certain rewards. Support and caring from significant others and symbolic parental figures is usually forthcoming. The patient usually is relieved of responsibilities as well as the expectations of others. If an individual has anxieties about his or her ability to fulfill these responsibilities and expectations, a factitious physical disorder may appear to be an attractive strategy. Thus, the disorder may represent a form of psychological coping similar in some functions to the somatoform disorders.

Conclusion

Factitious physical disorders represent a unique attempt by the individual to cope with the world. Once the physician gains some understanding of the disorder, the door is opened to therapeutic interventions that will allow the individual to cope more effectively. Management strategies are discussed in Chapter 11.

References

Aduan RP, Fauci AS, Dale DD, et al: Factitious fever and self induced infection. Ann Intern Med 90:230–242, 1979

Anderson PW, Galmarini M, Vagnucci A, et al: Factitious Cushing's disease. West J Med 159:487–489, 1993

American Psychiatric Association: Diagnostic and Statistical Manual of Mental Disorders, 4th Edition. Washington, DC, American Psychiatric Association, 1994, p 745

Apfelbaum JD, Williams HJ: Factitious simulation of systemic lupus erythematosus. West J Med 160:259–261, 1994

Asher R: Munchausen's syndrome. Lancet 1:339–341, 1951

Barker LH, Howell RJ: Munchausen syndrome by proxy in false allegations of child sexual abuse: legal implications. Bull Am Acad Psychiatry Law 22:499–510, 1994

Bialer PA, Wallack JJ: Mixed factitious disorder presenting as AIDS. Hosp Community Psychiatry 41:552–553, 1990

Churchill DR, De Cock KM, Miller RF: Feigned HIV infection/AIDS: malingering and Munchausen's syndrome. Genitourin Med 70:314–316, 1994

Cohen LM, Shapiro E, Manson JE, et al: The high cost of treating a psychiatric disorder as a medical/surgical illness. Psychosomatics 26:453–455, 1985

Cramer B, Gershberg MR, Stern M: Munchausen syndrome. Its relationship to malingering, hysteria, and the physician-patient relationship. Arch Gen Psychiatry 24:573–578, 1971

Duffy TP: The Red Baron. N Engl J Med 327:408–411, 1992

Earle JR, Folks DG: Factitious disorder and coexisting depression: a report of successful psychiatric consultation and case management. Gen Hosp Psychiatry 8:448–450, 1986

Eisendrath SJ: Factitious illness: a clarification. Psychosomatics 25:110–117, 1984

Eisendrath SJ: Factitious disorders and malingering, in Treatment of Psychiatric Disorders, 2nd Edition. Edited by Gabbard GO. Washington, DC, American Psychiatric Press, 1995a

Eisendrath SJ: Psychiatric aspects of chronic pain. Neurology 45:S26–S34, 1995b

Feldman MD, Escalona R: The longing for nurturance: a case of factitious cancer. Psychosomatics 32:226–227, 1991

Feldman MD, Ford CV: Patient or Pretender: Inside the Strange World of Factitious Disorders. New York, Wiley, 1994, pp 193–206

Folks DG: Munchausen's syndrome and other factitious disorders. Neurol Clin 13:267–281, 1995

Folks DG, Houck CA: Somatoform disorders, factitious disorders, and malingering, in Psychiatric Care of the Medical Patient. Edited by Stoudemire A, Fogel B. New York, Oxford University Press, 1993, pp 267–287

Ford CV: Lies! Lies!! Lies!!! The Psychology of Deceit. Washington, DC, American Psychiatric Press, 1996, pp 133–137

Folks DG, Freeman AM: Munchausen's syndrome and other factitious illness. Psychiatr Clin North Am 8:263–278, 1985

Ford CV: Munchausen syndrome, in Extraordinary Disorders of Human Behavior. Edited by Friedmann CTH, Faguet RA. New York, Plenum, 1982, pp 15–27

Ford CV: The Munchausen syndrome: a report of four new cases and a review of psychodynamic considerations. Int J Psychiatry Med 4:31–45, 1973

Ford CV, King BH, Hollender MH: Lies and liars: psychiatric aspects of prevarication. Am J Psychiatry 145:554–562, 1988

Ford CV, Stein R, Kelly MP, et al: Factitious aplastic anemia. J Nerv Ment Dis 172:369–372, 1984

Fras I, Coughlin BE: The treatment of factitious disease. Psychosomatics 12:117–122, 1971

Freyberger H, Nordmeyer JP, Freyberger HJ, et al: Patients suffering from factitious disorders in the clinico-psychosomatic consultation liaison service: psychodynamic processes, psychotherapeutic initial care and clinicointerdisciplinary cooperation. Psychother Psychosom 62:108–122, 1994

Gault MH, Campbell NR, Aksu AE: Spurious stones. Nephron 48:274–279, 1988

Gavin H: On Feigned and Factitious Diseases. Edinburgh, University Press, 1838, p 54

Geracioti TD, Van Dyke C, Mueller J, et al: The onset of Munchausen's syndrome. Gen Hosp Psychiatry 9:405–409, 1987

Herzberg JH, Wolff SM: Chronic factitious fever in puberty and adolescence. A diagnostic challenge to the family physician. Psychiatr Med 3:205–211, 1972

Ifudu O, Kolasinski SL, Friedman EA: Kidney-related Munchausen's syndrome. N Engl J Med 327:388–389, 1992

Kailasam MT, Parmer RJ, Stone RA, et al: Factitious pheochromocytoma: novel mimickry by Valsalva maneuver and clues to diagnosis. Am J Hypertens 8:651–655, 1995

Keiser HR: Surreptitious self-administration of epinephrine resulting in "pheochromocytoma." JAMA 266:1553–1555, 1991

Knockaert DC, Vanneste LJ, Vanneste SB, et al: Fever of unknown origin in the 1980s. An update of the diagnostic spectrum. Arch Intern Med 152:51–55, 1992

Nadelson T: The Munchausen spectrum: borderline character features. Gen Hosp Psychiatry 1:11–17, 1979

Nickl P: The Wonderful Travels and Adventures of Baron Munchhausen as Told by Himself in the Company of his Friends, and Washed Down by Many a Good Bottle of Wine. New York, North-South Books, 1992

Nordmeyer JP: An internist's view of patients with factitious disorders and factitious clinical symptomatology. Psychother Psychosom 62:30–40, 1994

Overholser JC: Differential diagnosis of malingering and factitious disorder with physical symptoms. Behav Sci Law 8:55–65, 1990

Pilowsky I: A general classification of abnormal illness behaviours. Br J Med Psychol 51:131–137, 1978

Powell R, Boast N: The Million Dollar Man: resource implications for chronic Munchausen's syndrome. Br J Psychiatry 162:253–256, 1993

Rand DC: Munchausen syndrome by proxy: a complex type of emotional abuse responsible for some false allegations of child abuse in divorce. Issues in Child Abuse Accusations 5:135–155, 1993

Reich P, Gottfried LA: Factitious disorders in a teaching hospital. Ann Intern Med 99:240–247, 1983

Rumans LW, Vosti KL: Factitious and fraudulent fever. Am J Med 65:745–755, 1978

Scully C, Eveson JW, Porter SR: Munchausen's syndrome: oral presentations. Br Dent J 21:65–67, 1995

Songer DA: Factitious AIDS: a case report and literature review. Psychosomatics 36:406–411, 1995

Spivak H, Rodin G, Sutherland A: The psychology of factitious disorders: a reconsideration. Psychosomatics 35:25–34, 1994

Stone MH: Factitious illness: psychological findings and treatment recommendations. Bull Menninger Clin 41:239–254, 1977

Taylor S, Hyler SE: Update on factitious disorders. Int J Psychiatry Med 23:81–94, 1993

Teasell RW, Shapiro AP: Strategic-behavioral intervention in the treatment of chronic nonorganic motor diagnosis. Am J Phys Med Rehabil 73:44–50, 1994

Topazian M, Binder HJ: Brief report: factitious diarrhea detected by measurement of stool osmolality. N Engl J Med 330:1418–1419, 1994

Wallach J: Laboratory diagnosis of factitious disorders. Arch Intern Med 154:1690–1696, 1994

CHAPTER 3

Factitious Psychological Disorders

Pamela E. Parker, M.D.

Psychological symptoms have always stymied the physician who depends on concrete evidence, such as laboratory values, for diagnosis. If a patient complains of general weakness, it is easier to assess for anemia than it is to question the validity of the complaint. Thus, in the area of factitious disorders, patients who present with psychological symptoms are a unique challenge, even for the physician who may be alert for factitious phenomena. In this chapter, the author provides a perspective on factitial psychological disorders within the spectrum of factitious disorders and illuminates aspects of the disorder that inform management.

Definition

According to DSM-IV (American Psychiatric Association 1994), the psychological subtype of factitious disorder is termed *Factitious Disorder With Predominantly Psychological Signs and Symptoms.* It states that

> This [psychological] subtype describes a clinical presentation in which psychological signs and symptoms predominate. It is characterized by the intentional production or feigning of psychological (often psychotic) symptoms that are suggestive of a mental disorder. . . . The presentation usually represents the individual's concept of mental disorder and may not conform to any recognized diagnostic category. (p. 47)

By circumscribing a subset of factitious disorders in this way, we are able to identify a hazy spot in the spectrum of factitious disorders. Thus, the DSM-IV distinction between factitious physical and factitious psychological disorders serves as a convenience but not always a clarification. Just as one cannot identify the point at which red becomes orange in the rainbow, one cannot identify the exact point at which physical symptoms become psychological.

For example, the report by Dohn (1986) of factitious rape illustrates the subtle nature of this spectrum concept. The patient has both physical and psychological symptomatology, as do several of the patients with factitious rape reported by Feldman et al. (1994). Although the complaint is clearly related to a physical violation, the patient gives a strong indication that the real difficulties lie in the psychological arena, and suggest posttraumatic stress disorder (PTSD).

The literature does not lack for discussions of the definitional complexities of factitious psychological disorders. These discussions have continued over the years (e.g., Gavin 1838) with attempts to clarify the murky issues. Merrin et al. (1986), for example, argued that factitious psychological and physical disorders should not be split into separate disorders but should merely carry a modifying statement to a unitary diagnostic code. Rogers et al. (1989) went even further, questioning whether factitious psychological disorders have any diagnostic legitimacy at all.

Regardless, the distinction of psychological from physical is becoming increasingly artificial in the face of neurophysiologic advances pointing to the interplay between psychology and neurobiology. If explanations of behavior are increasingly evident in terms of neurotransmitters, the distinctions between physical and psychological factitious disorders may best serve as indicators for treatment directions, which may include pharmacotherapy as well as behavioral modification and psychotherapy.

Epidemiology

As noted in Chapter 2, the incidence of factitious disorder is extremely difficult to measure because of the patient's intended deception of the physician. In many cases, the diagnosis is completely missed. This difficulty is compounded when one seeks to separate patients with primarily psychological complaints from those with primarily physical ones. Only a handful of factitious disorder cases that contain psychological symptoms exclusive of physical symptoms have been reported. Because the patient with factitious disorder may well have Munchausen syndrome, including the tendency to wander from one medical facility to another and to change his or her name, patients who appear to have had exclusively psychological symptoms may also have had physical symptoms, as reported elsewhere in the literature.

Another complicating factor in the epidemiology of factitious disorder with psychological symptoms is the difficulty of distinguishing the disorder from other similar psychiatric syndromes. Further discussion of this issue appears later in the section on differential diagnosis. The enormous overlap between dissociation, other somatizing disorders, and psychological factitious disorders leaves epidemiologic investigators with a daunting task.

Nicholson and Roberts (1994) have provided a succinct summary of current knowledge about the prevalence of psychological factitious disorders. If their data are compiled, the prevalence of psychological factitious disorders is approximately 0.14% of inpatient psychiatric admissions.

Clinical Features

Patients with factitious psychological disorders sometimes become the quintessential Munchausen patients, relating the most vivid, exciting, and dramatic stories. Because these patients rely on verbal exchange to capture the attention of medical caregivers, they are notably skilled at presenting their histories. Complaints of bereavement, PTSD, rape, and psychosis all gain credibility when conveyed with emotion and "fight-or-flight" urgency. Thus, pseudologia fantastica may be more prominent in patients with psychological symptoms than physical symptoms, and some degree of pathological lying is nearly always present. When uncovered, the true history of the patient is usually found to contain some severe emotional trauma but one that differs from the trauma that the patient describes (Rothchild 1994). Table 3–1 provides a summary of representative reported cases of factitious psychological disorders.

Table 3–1. Representative cases of factitious psychological disorders

Authors	**Cases, *n***	Symptoms or disorder
Oldham 1974	1	Chronic pain
Gelenberg 1977	1	Depression
Cheng and Hummel 1978	2	Depression, psychosis
Snowden et al. 1978	12	Bereavement
Pope et al. 1982	9	Psychosis
Phillips et al. 1983	20	Bereavement
Sparr and Pankratz 1983	5	PTSD
Lynn and Belza 1984	7	PTSD
Merrin et al. 1986	3	PTSD, major depression, pain
Jones and Horrocks 1987	1	Amnesia
Silber 1987	2	Eating disorders
Bhugra 1988	4	Depression, PTSD, bereavement, psychosis
Caradoc-Davies 1988	1	Alcohol abuse, amnesia
Fishbain et al. 1988	1	Chronic pain
Nickoloff et al. 1989	1	Bipolar disorder, depression, bereavement
Pankratz 1990	3	PTSD
Feldman and Russell 1991	1	Hypersomnia
Fishbain et al. 1991	4	Chronic pain
Ballas 1992	1	Recurrent pain
Popli et al. 1992	3	PTSD, depression, psychosis
Federoff et al. 1992	3?	Paraphilias
Parker 1993	1	Depression, PTSD
Feldman and Ford 1994	4	Transsexualism, schizophrenia, bereavement
Rothchild 1994	5	Bereavement
Songer 1995	1	Schizophrenia, depression
Neal and Rose 1995	1	PTSD
Feldman 1995	1	Dissociative identity disorder

Note. PTSD = posttraumatic stress disorder.

Beyond the greater flair with which the history is given, the characteristics of patients with factitious psychological symptoms are similar to those of patients with physical symptoms; this finding is not surprising, because the two classifications of symptoms are often found in the same patient. These patients feign symptomatology and, in severe forms, are peripatetic and deeply engrossed in the "con" game. Deception of the physician is paramount, and control issues (over caregivers and others) usually emerge. As with patients with factitious physical symptoms, patients with factitious psychological disorders tend to discharge themselves from the hospital if confronted. Patient history often indicates alcohol or drug abuse; in cases in which drug-seeking is the motivation for admission, the diagnosis of malingering is more accurate (see Case 1 presented later in this chapter).

As with physical factitious disorders, the symptoms may be more pronounced when the physician and hospital staff are present. If the patient is willing to provide valid psychological testing, traits of psychopathic deviation, paranoia, hysteria, depression, and hypochondriasis may be present (Bhugra 1988; Parker 1993).

That patients with falsified psychological symptoms are willing to accept psychiatric hospitalization offers perhaps the most clear distinction between patients with factitious physical symptoms and patients with factitious psychological symptoms. A common pattern for the factitious patient with physical symptoms is to leave the hospital against medical advice when referred to the psychiatric unit; the patient with factitious psychological symptoms, however, seeks hospitalization on the psychiatric unit. These patients may be steps closer to successful treatment than their counterparts with physical symptoms because they acknowledge the need for mental health care. If the physician understands that the factual content of a particular patient's complaints may be tainted but still addresses the distress of the patient, there is more likely to be a response to intervention. In contrast, patients with factitious physical symptoms are generally unable to discuss their feelings and thus may be much less amenable to addressing their internal distress.

Psychodynamics

The psychodynamic underpinnings in given cases of factitious disorder are often elusive, which contributes to the diagnostic imprecision many researchers perceive. Nevertheless, various theories have been espoused to account for the details of individual cases. These theories are no different for factitious disorder with psychological symptoms from what they are when physical symptoms predominate. The possibility that the patient needs to feel in control of authority figures—perhaps arising from the need for mastery over abusive parents—has been raised in numerous articles. More broadly, Hyler and Spitzer (1978) have suggested that the patient may be "attempting to gain mastery over a previously experienced psychic trauma," though O'Shea (1984) suggests that such theorizing may arise more from the physician's countertransference (e.g., a need to understand) than from reality. The longing for nurturing and the need for distraction from authentic life stressors are also motivation for deception in the medical setting.

Detection

Psychological symptoms lack the biologic markers that might be available in the factitious physical disorder patient. Thus, the diagnosis of factitious disorder with purely psychological symptoms can be much more difficult than the diagnosis of factitious physical disorder.

For a number of reasons, the physician is especially inclined to believe the patient with falsified psychological symptoms. One reason is that psychological symptoms still are associated with stigma, which often leads the physician to believe that a patient with mental complaints is unlikely to feign these to serve a hidden agenda. Another reason is that the physician has no indication that what the patient is saying is not true. In a busy emergency room, for instance, symptoms of depression or claims of bereavement are rarely questioned. In addition, the resources needed to confirm psychosocial data are not nearly as available as the laboratory is for obtaining physiologic data. Finally, physicians and staff members in acute care settings are often not as familiar with the processes of obtaining information from social networks as they are from other medical facilities.

Thus, to arrive at the proper diagnosis, the physician and his or her staff must be alert to indications of deception that may be quite subtle. These clues are often buried in the discrepancy between what the patient says and his or her actual appearance or behavior. For example, in a case reported elsewhere by the author (Parker 1993), the patient—who had a documented depression and increasing suicidal behavior for one month prior to admission—was found to be wearing chartreuse nail polish, a choice out of character for a patient with apparent depression. The presence of symptomatology of Ganser's syndrome (Ganser 1965), especially the phenomenon of *vorbeireden* or "approximate answers" (e.g., Examiner: "What is two plus two?"; Patient: "Five"), was then elicited only because of an elevated index of suspicion. Similarly, the patient in the following case report was noted to be wearing brightly colored clothing and to demonstrate cheerful affect while describing the symptoms of depression. Though these findings do not in and of themselves negate the diagnosis of depression, they are warnings that the physician should look carefully for other inconsistencies or, as stated by Oldham (1974), "a deficit in the patient's credibility."

Diagnosis and treatment in factitious psychological disorder are often carried out concurrently, as is the case with many medical disorders (e.g., when a brain tumor is removed and pathologic analysis can then be performed). Thus, the patient with factitious disorder with psychological symptoms may require cautious evaluation in order not to exacerbate his or her pathology. Eisendrath (1984) has cautioned against a heavy-handed confrontational approach.

There are a number of clues that commonly arise in factitious psychological disorder cases. First, the patient is unlikely to have many visitors, either because friends and relatives have been alienated or because they might reveal the true nature of the patient's difficulty. Second, the patient is unlikely to present with classic findings of a psychiatric disorder; as noted, the patient's symptoms will instead typically represent his or her concept of the mental disorder. It appears that patients with factitious psychological disorders are less likely to have had medical or psychiatric training than those with factitious physical symptoms, and, therefore, they will have "learned" their symptoms from the media, previous hospitalization, or other life experiences. Third, use of pharmacologic interventions may prove futile; medications indicated for the condition the patient is feigning may appear inexplicably ineffective. Such surprising pharmacologic failures can be especially important clues to the diagnosis.

Differential Diagnosis

The patient may, in fact, have the very disorder that she or he is attempting to simulate. The patient previously reported by Parker (1993), for example, was admitted to the hospital for depression and suicidal behavior. She also presented with symptoms and signs of dementia and delirium and could have been diagnosed with dissociative disorder not otherwise specified, PTSD, and/or pseudodementia. After the patient's background was elucidated, the possibility of dissociative identity disorder (multiple personality disorder) was added to the differential diagnosis. Although the content of virtually all of the material the patient gave was discovered to have been fabricated, she nonetheless eventually proved partially responsive to psychotherapy and an antidepressant. This response partially validated one of the diagnoses—major depression—that she had been attempting to simulate.

In other cases, the patient's simulation of a mental disorder may actually be the prodrome to an authentic mental disorder with a serious outcome, as suggested by Nicholson and Roberts (1994) and Pope et al. (1982). Rogers et al. (1989) urge caution when diagnosing factitious psychosis because a number of these patients eventually manifest clear-cut psychotic disorders such as schizophrenia.

In DSM-IV, Ganser's syndrome is presented as an example of dissociative disorder not otherwise specified. At various times, however, it was considered to fall within the realm of factitious disorders with psychological symptoms. The hallmark of Ganser's syndrome is approximate answers, illustrated previously, but the literature contains an impressive variety of accompanying symptomatology. Amnesia, disorientation, and hallucinations are each found in at least half of the reported cases of Ganser's syndrome (Cocores 1984). Although the syndrome has been shown to be present in some patients with impaired cognitive abilities and previous brain injury, there is clearly some conscious component to the responses provided by the patient, because random answers would not be approximate. Early reports of Ganser's syndrome involved prisoners (Ganser 1965), raising the notion that the syndrome functioned to achieve the external gain of escape from a noxious situation. These reports also suggested that the presence of approximate answers placed the diagnosis closer to frank malingering than dissociative or conversion disorders. Other authors, however, who described Ganser's syndrome in settings such as general hospitals (Weiner and Braiman 1955), suggested that approximate answers occur in some forms of pseudodementia or depression; if so, the syndrome would be primarily an unconscious phenomenon more accurately identified as a conversion disorder.

Other dissociative disorders also must be considered in the differential diagnosis of factitious disorders. Dissociative fugue and dissociative identity disorder may result in alterations of memory and inconsistent factual information. In the author's case mentioned previously (Parker 1993), the possibility of dissociative identity disorder was not seriously considered until approximately 1 year after the patient's discharge from the hospital. As the patient became more involved in psychotherapy, she spent a number of sessions sitting in absolute silence. During her second year of psychotherapy, she began to suggest in one session that she had "other names" and might be other ages. Although the author considered the possibility that these statements and behaviors indicated an authentic dissociative disorder, her new symptoms were given no more of the physician's attention than any other potential attention-seeking behaviors had been given in the past. The complaints of multiple names and personalities disappeared within a short time, as did many other sensational complaints that she had produced. Because the patient's history suggested that significant sexual abuse had indeed occurred, the author remained alert to the possible reemergence of these symptoms, but they did not recur during ongoing therapy.

The subtleties of classification can be beguiling whenever the diagnostician is called upon to determine the degree of consciousness of motivation (Cunnien 1988), a task that commonly arises when distinguishing malingering from factitious disorder. The following case demonstrates this conundrum:

Case 1

An unmarried young woman visited her family physician many times over a 6-month period. She complained of vague, migrating neurologic symptoms, ultimately prompting extensive laboratory measures to rule out multiple sclerosis. When the evaluation

> proved negative for any pathology, the patient began to complain of depression. As she discussed her depression, she revealed a number of sexual encounters. Her family physician, attentive to the many features of somatization in the patient's medical history, sought the assistance of a psychiatrist. The family physician and the psychiatrist agreed to see the patient separately on the same day.
>
> On the day of the appointments, the patient was seen first by the family physician. She was wearing a dress of brilliant red, gold, and purple. As the family physician brought the interview to a close and started to leave the room, the patient turned to him and said, "If you weren't married, I would have the 'hots' for you."
>
> The evaluation by the psychiatrist offered little objective evidence for a depressive disorder. Review of the chart, reinforced by findings during subsequent visits, confirmed that the patient had contrived her physical and psychological complaints to see the family physician, to whom she was attracted. During future visits with this patient, the family doctor asked for a nurse to be present, and the patient summarily dropped out of his care. It was subsequently discovered that the patient had sought the care of another young male physician in the community, to whom she had also made comments containing sexual innuendos.

This case demonstrates the difficulty of attempting to demarcate factitious psychological disorder and malingering. As described by Feldman and Escalona (1991), the need for nurturing is powerful, and this motivation tends to point toward a diagnosis of factitious disorder; however, sexual impulses can be powerful as well, and the pursuit of a desired sex partner through fabricated depression suggests malingering. Assessment and comparison of all the motivations leading to a particular behavior, and the extent to which each is conscious or unconscious, may be an elusive task for even the most sophisticated evaluator. Often the diagnosis can be made only in retrospect, and even then it is difficult to place it precisely within the spectrum of abnormal illness behavior. The diagnosis in Case 1 remains unclear. The patient's history contained sufficient childhood stressors to warrant the need for nurturing. On the other hand, her frank desire for a sexual relationship could be considered an obvious secondary gain.

Conclusion

The distinction between factitious psychological and factitious physical disorders is complex. On the one hand, it is helpful to distinguish sets of patients that behave somewhat differently from one another. On the other hand, these patients' motivations seem to be the same, and separation of the psychological from the physical can be artificial, ignoring the interplay between these two domains.

The current classification of factitious disorders has helped to clarify the terminology to be used when an unconsciously produced disorder is stimulated by unconscious motivation (conversion disorder) and when a consciously produced disorder is stimulated by conscious motivation (malingering). However, enormous difficulty persists in distinguishing the conscious from unconscious in a practical sense. These struggles emerge even more urgently in cases of suspected factitious psychological disorders. (Treatment issues are discussed in Chapter 11.)

References

American Psychiatric Association: Diagnostic and Statistical Manual of Mental Disorders, 4th Edition. Washington, DC, American Psychiatric Association, 1994

Ballas SK: Munchausen sickle cell painful crisis. Annals of Clinical and Laboratory Science 22:226–228, 1992

Bhugra D: Psychiatric Munchausen's syndrome. Acta Psychiatr Scand 77:497–503, 1988

Caradoc-Davies G: Feigned alcohol abuse. Br J Psychiatry 152:418–420, 1988

Cheng L, Hummel L: The Munchausen syndrome as a psychiatric condition. Br J Psychiatry 133:20–21, 1978

Cocores JA, Santa WG, Patel MD: The Ganser syndrome: evidence suggesting its classification as a dissociative disorder. Int J Psychiatry Med 14:47–56, 1984

Cunnien AJ: Psychiatric and medical syndromes associated with deception, in Clinical Assessment of Malingering and Deception. Edited by Rogers R. New York, Guilford, 1988, pp 13–33

Dohn HH: Factitious rape: a case report. Hillside J Clin Psychiatry 8:224–231, 1986

Eisendrath SJ: Factitious illness: a clarification. Psychosomatics 25:110–117, 1984

Fedoroff JP, Hanson A, McGuire M, et al: Simulated paraphilias: a preliminary study of patients who imitate or exaggerate paraphilic symptoms and behaviors. J Forensic Sci 37:902–911, 1992

Feldman MD: Factitious Munchausen's syndrome: a confession. N Engl J Med 327:438–439, 1992

Feldman MD: Illness or illusion?: distinguishing malingering and factitious disorder. Primary Psychiatry 2:39–41, 1995

Feldman MD, Escalona R: The longing for nurturance: a case of factitious cancer. Psychosomatics 32:226–228, 1991

Feldman MD, Ford CV: Patient or Pretender: Inside the Strange World of Factitious Disorders. New York, Wiley, 1994, pp 130–145

Feldman MD, Russell JL: Factitious cyclic hypersomnia: a new variant of factitious disorder. South Med J 84:379–381, 1991

Feldman MD, Ford CV, Stone T: Deceiving others/deceiving oneself: four cases of factitious rape. South Med J 87:736–738, 1994

Fishbain DA, Goldberg M, Rosomoff RS, et al: Munchausen syndrome presenting with chronic pain: case report. Pain 35:91–94, 1988

Folks DG, Freeman AM III: Munchausen's syndrome and other factitious illness. Psychiatr Clin North Am 8:263–278, 1985

Ganser SJM: A peculiar hysterical state. Translated by Schorer CE. British Journal of Criminology 5:120–126, 1965

Gavin H: On Feigned and Factitious Diseases. Edinburgh, University Press, 1838, pp 51–83

Gelenberg AJ: Munchausen's syndrome with a psychiatric presentation. Diseases of the Nervous System 38:378–380, 1977

Hyler SE, Spitzer RL: Hysteria split asunder. Am J Psychiatry 135:1500–1504, 1978

Jones JR, Horrocks FA: Fictitious epilepsy associated with amnesia. Br J Psychiatry 150:257–258, 1987

Lynn EJ, Belza M: Factitious posttraumatic stress disorder: the veteran who never got to Vietnam. Hosp Community Psychiatry 35:697–701, 1984

McDowell CP: Suicide disguised as murder: a dimension of Munchausen syndrome. J Forensic Sci 32:254–261, 1987

Mehl AL, Coble L, Johnson S: Munchausen syndrome by proxy: a family affair. Child Abuse Negl 14:577–585, 1990

Merrin EL, van Dyke C, Cohen S, et al: Dual factitious disorder. Gen Hosp Psychiatry 8:246–250, 1986

Neal LA, Rose MC: Factitious post traumatic stress disorder: a case report. Med Sci Law 35:352–354, 1995

Nicholson SD, Roberts GA: Patients who (need to) tell stories. Br J Hosp Med 51:546–549, 1994

Nickoloff SE, Neppe VM, Ries RK: Factitious AIDS. Psychosomatics 30:342–345, 1989

Oldham L: Facial pain as a presentation in von Munchausen's syndrome: a case report. Br J Oral Maxillofac Surg 12:68–90, 1974

O'Shea B: More on patients with factitious illness. Am J Psychiatry 141:140–141, 1984

Pankratz L: Continued appearance of factitious posttraumatic stress disorder. Am J Psychiatry 147:811–812, 1990

Parker PE: A case of Munchausen syndrome with psychological symptoms. Psychosomatics 34:360–364, 1993

Phillips MR, Ward NG, Ries RK: Factitious mourning: painless patienthood. Am J Psychiatry 140:420–425, 1983

Pope HG Jr, Jonas JM, Jones B: Factitious psychosis: phenomenology, family history and long-term outcome of nine patients. Am J Psychiatry 139:1480–1483, 1982

Popli AP, Masand PS, Dewan MJ: Factitious disorders with psychological symptoms. J Clin Psychiatry 53:325–328, 1992

Rogers R, Bagby RM, Rector N: Diagnostic legitimacy of factitious disorder with psychological symptoms. Am J Psychiatry 146:1312–1314, 1990

Rothchild E: Fictitious twins, factitious illness. Psychiatry 57:326–332, 1994

Shelly WB: Dermatitis artefacta induced in a patient by one of her multiple personalities. Br J Dermatology 105:587–589, 1981

Silber TJ: Acquired pseudo eating disorder. J Adolesc Health Care 8:452–455, 1987

Snowdon J, Solomons R, Druce H: Feigned bereavement: twelve cases. Br J Psychiatry 133:15–19, 1978

Songer DA: Factitious AIDS: a case report and literature review. Psychosomatics 36:406–411, 1995

Sparr L, Pankratz LD: Factitious posttraumatic stress disorder. Am J Psychiatry 140:1016–1019, 1983

Weiner H, Braiman A: The Ganser syndrome. Am J Psychiatry 111:767–773, 1955

CHAPTER 4

Ethical and Legal Issues in Factitious Disorders: An Overview

Charles V. Ford, M.D.

Patients who have or are suspected to have factitious disorders create unique ethical and medicolegal issues for physicians and other health care professionals. In the past, the rights of these patients have often been ignored. Recent case reports, however, suggest that such attitudes not only are countertherapeutic but may also precipitate medicolegal conflicts; these patients can and do retain attorneys and initiate malpractice suits.

This overview is intended to provide clinicians, particularly psychiatrists, with insight into the various ethical and medicolegal issues that may be anticipated when they encounter patients with factitious disorders. In this chapter, the author offers recommendations for appropriate interventions. For didactic purposes, ethical and medicolegal matters are addressed separately, but in real life they are often richly intertwined.

Ethical Issues

The doctor-patient relationship becomes problematic when it involves willful deceit by the patient. The physician, after learning of such deceit, may react with anger or vindictiveness that has the effect of undermining any potential therapeutic progress. The following ethical issues are among the most salient that have been identified.

Confidentiality

The principle of confidentiality in the doctor-patient relationship dates back to the Hippocratic Oath. The American Medical Association's (AMA) first code of medical ethics (1847/1977) describes the physician's obligation to secrecy as absolute except when it is *imperative* to violate it. The converse of this requirement was the stated duty of patients to communicate faithfully and unreservedly to their physicians about the supposed cause of their ailments. However, in 1957, the AMA modified its prior stance, limiting the potential relinquishment of confidentiality only to situations in which the physician "is required to do so by law or unless it becomes necessary in order to protect the welfare of the individual or of the community." The more restrictive Declaration of Geneva of the World Medical Association (1977) did not legitimize any violations of confidentiality.

Ethical dilemmas are created when two principles are in conflict. This situation occurs frequently with factitious disorders because the preservation of confidentiality demanded by a patient may well prove harmful to other persons or even the patient him- or herself. In a case published by Ford and Abernethy (1981), this dilemma is highlighted. A young woman, through surreptitiously self-induced disease, was ruining her husband's career because of the demands made upon him for her care. When the diagnosis of factitious disorder was finally established, the patient expressly forbade the psychiatric consultant to communicate this information to either her husband or her primary care doctor. Thus, the consultant was faced with the dilemma that honoring confidentiality, a valued principle, would also permit the factitious behavior to continue, with destructive consequences to another party (the patient's husband), to the patient herself, and to the community through the costs of her medical care.

Resolution of this type of conundrum can be argued in different ways. A utilitarian approach would favor acting in a way that produces the greatest good for the greatest number of persons; viewed in this way, violation of confidentiality would be justified in this case. A contrasting perspective would hold that the compromise of principles often starts one on a "slippery slope" and is, in the long run, destructive to the basic foundations of medical care; from such a perspective, disclosure would be opposed.

The argument has sometimes been made that, in the case of factitious disease, the perpetrator is a miscreant who, because of deceit, does not fulfill the part of the contract with caregivers that establishes patienthood. Thus, if no genuine doctor-patient relationship exists, then the physician is not bound by the code of ethics (Ford and Zaner 1987; Meropol et al. 1985). Indeed, "blacklists" of patients with factitious disorder have been proposed in many countries for distribution to health care providers, and they are apparently in use in Australia (Mohammed et al. 1985). In the United States, however, the use of such lists has been firmly discouraged because of ethical considerations, the potential for medicolegal liability, and ineffectiveness (Kass 1985).

Irrespective of alternative intellectual arguments, the conservative course of action is for the physician to honor confidentiality except in clear-cut situations in which adherence to this policy would be harmful specifically to the patient and/or another party (Kass 1985). In such situations, a multidisciplinary task force (comprising physicians, nurses, social workers, hospital administrators, a hospital attorney, and, when available, an ethicist) can help shape policy and share responsibility for difficult decisions.

Invasion of Privacy

The medical literature is replete with descriptions of how the diagnosis of factitious disorder was made by searching a patient's belongings and finding paraphernalia such as syringes or concealed medications. Some authors have written with unmistakable pride of devising elaborate diagnostic procedures that have confirmed the factitious nature of the patient's illness. For example, in a case of factitious hypoglycemia reported by Berkowitz and colleagues (1971), physicians placed a radioactive isotope in vials of insulin a patient had concealed in her hospital room. Monitored the next day, the patient's slight radioactivity confirmed that she had injected herself with the insulin.

The present climate of medical practice has moved considerably away from the paternalism inherent in such approaches. There has been a sharply increased recognition of patients' rights. Not only do patients retain all civil rights on admission to a hospital, they also have the rights of informed consent and informed refusal; thus, no procedure should be initiated without the patient's knowledge and consent. Meropol and colleagues (1985) hold the position that searches or laboratory investigations without the full consent of a patient are unethical. Instead, when factitious behavior is suspected, the physician should first communicate to the patient that factitious disorder has been incorporated into the differential diagnosis, then request permission for further exploration of that possibility. Opponents can argue that allowing such a patient to continue to self-induce disease may lead to disability or death; in such an eventuality, the patient's autonomy would be compromised even more conspicuously than if a secret search were mounted. However, similar arguments, if extrapolated, would favor the abolition of patient choice regarding smoking cigarettes, drinking alcohol, or riding motorcycles.

Misuse of Scarce Resources

The patient with a factitious disease uses an enormous quantity of medical care in terms of time and expense. On occasion, scarce biologic resources are misappropriated as well (e.g., HLA-matched platelets [Ford et al. 1984]). Once the diagnosis of factitious disease is established, what is the obligation to permit the misuse of these resources as well as the time of physicians and other health care personnel? To what extent must the physician continue care? Should caregivers who withdraw care under such circumstances be liable for abandonment? In theory, a physician, with appropriate notice to the patient, can withdraw from a case. However, a related question can be appropriately asked: What physician knowing of the factitious behavior would be willing to assume the care of such a patient (Sadler 1987)? As mentioned previously, the responsibility for difficult management decisions, as in this situation, is best shared. A multidisciplinary group might carefully evaluate the specifics of an individual case and render an opinion that guides the treatment plan and decisions about ongoing care.

One such case involved a 23-year-old nursing student who repeatedly presented nearly in coma to the emergency department of a large church-affiliated hospital. Her private internist, who had frequently been called out at night to care for her, determined that her hypoglycemic episodes were caused by surreptitious injections of insulin. Frustrated and angry, he requested a "curbside" psychiatric consultation. The consultant recommended a meeting to include the internist, personnel from the emergency department, social service representatives, and the hospital chaplain.

As a result of the meeting, the attendees suggested that the internist and facility continue to offer medical care to the patient, despite her refusal of psychiatric treatment. However, they held that this care should be rendered in a matter-of-fact style that did not require the internist to respond personally to every instance of hypoglycemia. With the patient now unable to perpetuate the drama of the previous episodes or to "split" the staff, the number of hypoglycemic episodes was markedly reduced.

Medicolegal Issues

Involuntary Hospitalization or Treatment

The patient with factitious disorder is often engaged in self-destructive behavior that leads to permanent maiming or even death (Nichols et al. 1990; Sutherland and Rodin 1990). Such a patient might benefit from court-mandated treatment or some other form of protection from him- or herself. Experience with involuntary treatment of factitious disorder is limited, and the laws of most states may not be sufficiently flexible to provide for commitment. In an unusual case in Alabama (Houck 1992), a woman who had already destroyed one kidney and continued to self-infect her genitourinary system was committed to a state hospital for her protection. Unfortunately, the psychiatrist at this overworked facility declared that her condition was "not treatable," and she was discharged after several days. Still, two other case reports do indicate that extended involuntary hospitalization resulted in some progress regarding the patients' propensities with factitious behavior (Miller et al. 1985; Yassa 1978).

The use of an outpatient guardianship to manage and limit a Munchausen syndrome patient's abuse of medical facilities was described by McFarland and colleagues (1983). These authors believed that the use of a public guardian to monitor and provide consent for medical procedures would be more palatable to the judge than civil commitment because the Oregon guardianship statutes were less precisely drawn. This particular legal tactic may have the potential for wider use, particularly if a patient can be restricted from traveling to other states for medical intervention.

Prosecution for Fraudulent Abuse of Medical Services

Few states have enacted legislation against the fraudulent acquisition of medical services (Lipsitt 1982). Such behavior, if not recompensed, can be viewed as the stealing of the time and expertise of health care professionals and abuse of other resources (Ford and Zaner 1989). As factitious disorders become better known, it is possible that laws governing this type of behavior will become more widespread. In a case in Arizona, for example, a patient was prosecuted for fraud associated with psychiatric, medical, and dental services, and she ultimately pled guilty (Feldman 1995).

Malpractice Liability

Physicians and other health care professionals may feel secure that they are immune to lawsuits filed by patients with factitious disorders. They may reason that, considering the patient's culpability in deceiving others, they could not possibly be held accountable for any medical consequences. However, caregivers should not feel secure. Despite the patients' outrageous behaviors perpetrating a variety of fraudulent acts, some individuals with factitious disorders do initiate lawsuits (Feldman and Ford 1994; Lipsitt 1986). These suits, considered at greater length in Chapter 5, generally incorporate one of two tactics.

One tactic is for the patient to deny any factitious behavior and sue for an apparent untoward response to a procedure, though, in reality, the patient may have self-induced the response. In one such case, a patient with borderline personality disorder became infatuated with (i.e., "idealized") her surgeon. She was able to maintain her relationship with him by infecting her surgical wound with feces. Later, when she became angry at the doctor for imagined rejection (i.e., "devalued" him), she retaliated by initiating a lawsuit. Rather than the expected vindication for the physician, the initial lawsuit resulted in a hung jury because jurors could not believe that a nonpsychotic person could infect herself with feces (Feldman and Ford 1994). As explained in Chapter 5, when patients with feigned or self-induced illnesses enter the legal setting, the dividing line between the terms *malingering* and *factitious disorder* becomes unclear (Ford 1992; Jonas and Pope 1985).

A second tactic that a patient with factitious disorder can use in a malpractice suit is to claim negligence on the part of the physician to recognize and treat the factitious disorder itself (Lipsitt 1986). Within this scenario, any invasive procedures represent unwarranted assaults upon the patient that would have been avoided by a more astute clinician. Thus, the clinician is well advised to attend to the warning signs of factitious disorder early in the course of a diagnostic evaluation.

Factitious Disorder by Proxy (Munchausen Syndrome by Proxy)

Factitious disorder by proxy (FDP) introduces complexities into the ethical and legal issues faced by the physician that are more fully described in Chapter 8. In FDP, the physician has to attend not simply to one individual but rather to the interrelationships of two or more, including the perpetrator and his or her victims.

The DSM-IV diagnosis of factitious disorder not otherwise specified and the explicit use of FDP as an example of a phenomenon that could fulfill the corresponding criteria, now allows for an official diagnosis of FDP (American Psychiatric Association 1994). However, in the opinion of this author, the diagnosis of factitious disorder, not otherwise specified, when referring to FDP, should be reserved for the victim, not the perpetrator. Providing a formal psychiatric diagnosis for the perpetrator may allow for a defense on the basis of diminished responsibility (Sigal et al. 1990) because the behavior is related to a psychiatric disorder. Such defense arguments have already been made. This author believes that any psychiatric diagnosis assigned to perpetrators should be limited to those Axis I and Axis II categories for which they qualify, independently of the factitious behavior.

As an assault on the bodily and/or psychologic integrity of another individual, FDP is a crime. Though, as described elsewhere in this book, not all cases of induced factitious disease have involved an adult harming a child (e.g., Sigal et al. 1991; Sigal et al. 1990; Repper 1995; Yorker 1988), most FDP cases do involve parents (mostly mothers) inducing or simulating disease states in their children. As such, FDP has been recognized as a form of child abuse (Meadow 1977). Depending on several variables, including severity, child abuse may be dealt with by child protective agencies, juvenile or family courts, and/or criminal courts. Irrespective of which judicial jurisdiction ultimately may have responsibility for the case, however, it behooves the physician to conduct him- or herself in a manner that respects the needs and rights of the patient and suspected perpetrator. One must also remember that medical records, investigative procedures, and opinions will become a part of the legal process. Medicolegal issues related to FDP have been outlined by several authors (Houck 1992; Newberger 1992; Schreier and Libow 1993; Yorker and Kahan 1991) and are more fully described in Chapter 8. The following brief summary is offered as an overview.

FDP and the definition of child abuse. Abuse is defined (in the Child Abuse Prevention and Treatment Act of 1974, as cited by DeAngelis 1992) as "the physical and mental injuring, sexual abuse, negligent treatment or maltreatment of a child under the age of 18 by a person who is responsible for the child's welfare under circumstances which indicate that the child's health and welfare is harmed or threatened thereby. . . ." Clearly, FDP meets this definition of child abuse.

Reporting requirements. In all 50 states, there is a legal requirement, with penalties for a failure to comply, for physicians to report cases of suspected child abuse to child protective agencies (DeAngelis 1992). This legal requirement supersedes all claims to confidentiality insofar as the report is reasonable and made in good faith. Since FDP meets the definition of child abuse, there is a legal requirement to report suspected FDP cases. However, the authorities to whom such reports are made may need to be educated as to the nature of FDP. Even child advocates may initially react with disbelief that a mother could deliberately induce disease in her child.

Documentation. It is essential that careful medical records be maintained to document findings, including circumstantial evidence, that suggest FDP. For example, do symptoms remit when the mother is absent for a few hours or days? Other information that is important, perhaps vital, relates to a determination of a pattern to the medical contacts. Medical records for the patient and siblings, accessed from all possible sources, are important to obtain. The deaths of siblings during childhood is a particularly ominous piece of information (Bools et al. 1992).

Covert surveillance. When a mother or other caretaker is suspected of producing the patient's symptoms, no evidence is more powerful than direct observation of her illness-inducing acts. However, she is likely to constrain her abusive behavior if she believes she is being watched. For this reason, covert surveillance of the interactions between mother and child in the hospital has been advocated (British Paediatric Association 1994; Feldman 1994). Hidden video-camera observation of a child, for example, has provided conclusive evidence of maternal behaviors such as smothering the child or introducing toxic substances into his or her mouth (Samuels et al 1992). Yet, this technique is problematical from an ethical and medicolegal perspective because it may be regarded as an invasion of privacy or the obtaining of evidence through unlawful means (Evans 1995). On the other hand, to warn the mother that video surveillance is to begin may result in her flight, with the child, to another hospital where the child is again placed at risk. Meadow (1987) has observed that if the child were able to provide permission in these circumstances, he or she certainly would agree to it.

Placement of a hidden video camera and/or similar techniques should not be undertaken in a capricious manner. It should be preceded by discussions with the hospital staff and management, the hospital attorney, law enforcement authorities, and, if available, an ethics committee. Further, in view of the possibility that video surveillance will produce evidence of factitial disease behavior, it is necessary to have appropriate legal and/or psychiatric interventions prearranged. Epstein and colleagues (1987) have reported a carefully planned intervention that illustrates these considerations.

Expert testimony in FDP. The 1981 case of *People v. Phillips* (as cited by Yorker and Kahan 1991) was a legal landmark for the recognition of FDP as a variant of child abuse. In an action affirmed by the California Court of Appeals, expert testimony was allowed as to the phenomenon of FDP and the extent to which the defendant mother, Priscilla Phillips, fit the profile of a perpetrator. Expert testimony about FDP is now widely permitted. Of note, a legal precedent in federal courts, with later affirmation by the U.S. Supreme Court, allowed evidence to be introduced concerning the deaths of other siblings as well. This ruling was, in essence, a recognition that in cases of infanticide, the repetition of childhood demise in a single family not only may be relevant but also may be the only evidence necessary to prove the crime (DiMaio and Bernstein 1974).

At this time, there seems to be little doubt that FDP may be a serial activity involving multiple children and one that also places future children at risk (Alexander et al. 1990; Bools et al. 1992). Accurate detailed documentation at the time of hospitalization is essential (Rand 1989), because considerable time may pass between the suspected acts and court proceedings.

Conclusion

Management of the patient with a factitious disorder is notably difficult. Medical problems, complicated by an inaccurately reported history and continued surreptitious symptom production, require treatment. In the process of attending to these needs, the physicians and other health professionals face several potential ethical and medicolegal complexities. The time-consuming nature of these patients and their problems often elicit anger and the potential for caregivers to react in counterproductive ways (Houck 1992). The following guidelines are proposed in order to minimize iatrogenic complications to the management of these vexing patients:

- Factitious disorders should be considered, and often formally included, in the differential diagnosis of patients with poorly explained complaints, inconsistent laboratory findings, or failure to respond to treatment in a predictable manner.
- When factitious disorder or FDP is suspected, a multidisciplinary task force should be convened to consider the ethical and medicolegal issues in management. Participants optimally will

include psychiatrists and other physicians, nurses, social workers, hospital administrators, an attorney, and an ethicist.

- Persons with suspected or even confirmed factitious disorders continue to retain their civil rights with regard to privacy, confidentiality, and treatment. Any exception to these principles should clearly be in the best interests of the patient (e.g., the victim in cases of FDP) and preferably undertaken after consultation with the multidisciplinary task force described above.
- Suspicions of FDP (particularly involving a child) must be reported to the appropriate authorities.
- When factitious illness is suspected, careful documentation of all information, including that referable to siblings in cases of possible FDP, is essential and may be life-saving.

References

Alexander R, Smith W, Stevenson R: Serial Munchausen by proxy. Pediatrics 86:581–585, 1990

American Medical Association: Principles of medical ethics. JAMA 164:1484, 1957

American Medical Association: First code of medical ethics (1847). Reprinted from Proceedings of the National Medical Convention 1846–1847, in Ethics in Medicine: Historical Perspectives and Contemporary Concerns. Edited by Reiser SJ, Dyck AJ, Curran WL. Cambridge, MA, MIT Press, 1977

American Psychiatric Association: Diagnostic and Statistical Manual of Mental Disorders, 4th Edition. Washington, DC, American Psychiatric Association, 1994

Berkowitz S, Parrish JE, Field JB: Factitious hypoglycemia: why not diagnose before laparotomy. Am J Med 51:669–674, 1971

Bools CN, Neale BA, Meadow SR: Comorbidity associated with fabricated illness (Munchausen syndrome by proxy). Arch Dis Child 67:77–79, 1992

British Paediatric Association: Evaluation of suspected imposed upper airway obstruction. London, British Paediatric Association, 1994

DeAngelis C: Clinical indicators of child abuse, in Clinical Handbook of Child Psychiatry and the Law. Edited by Schetky DE, Benedek EP. Baltimore, MD, Williams & Wilkins, 1992, pp 104–118

DiMaio VJM, Bernstein CG: A case of infanticide. J Forensic Sci 19: 745–754, 1974

Epstein M, Markowitz RL, Gallo DM, et al: Munchausen syndrome by proxy: consideration in diagnosis and confirmation by video surveillance. Pediatrics 80:220–224, 1987

Evans D: The investigation of life-threatening child abuse and Munchausen syndrome by proxy. J Med Ethics 21:9–13, 1995

Feldman MD. Spying on mothers. Lancet 344:132, 1994

Feldman MD. Factitious disorders and fraud. Psychosomatics 36:509–510, 1995

Feldman MD, Ford CV: Patient or Pretender: Inside the Strange World of Factitious Disorders. New York, Wiley, 1994, pp 64, 94–95, 162

Ford CV: Illness as a lifestyle: the role of somatization in medical practice. Spine 17:S338–343, 1992

Ford CV, Abernethy V: Factitious illness: a multidisciplinary consideration of ethical issues. Gen Hosp Psychiatry 3:329–336, 1981

Ford CV, Stein RS, Kelly MP, et al: Factitial aplastic anemia. J Nerv Ment Dis 172:369–372, 1984

Ford CV, Zaner RM: Response to the article "Ethical and management considerations in factitious illness: one and the same" by John Z. Sadler. Gen Hosp Psychiatry 9:37–39, 1987

Houck CA: Medicolegal aspects of factitious disorder. Psychiatr Med 10:105–116, 1992

Jonas JM, Pope HG: The dissimulating disorders: a single diagnostic entity. Compr Psychiatry 26:58–62, 1985

Kass FC: Identification of persons with Munchausen's syndrome: ethical problems. Gen Hosp Psychiatry 7:195–200, 1985

Lipsitt DR: The enigma of factitious illness, in Medical and Health Annual. Chicago, Encyclopedia Britannica, 1982

Lipsitt DR: The factitious patient who sues. Am J Psychiatry 143:1482, 1986

McFarland BH, Resnick M, Bloom JD: Ensuring continuity of care for a Munchausen patient through a public guardian. Hosp Community Psychiatry 34:65–67, 1983

Meadow R: Munchausen syndrome by proxy: the hinterland of child abuse. Lancet 2:343–345, 1977

Meadow R: Video recording and child abuse. BMJ 294:1629–1630, 1987

Meropol NJ, Ford CV, Zaner RM: Factitious illness: an exploration in ethics. Perspect Biol Med 28:269–281, 1985

Miller RD, Blanck FW, Doren DM, et al: The Munchausen patient in a forensic facility. Psychiatr Q 57:72–76, 1985

Mohammed R, Goy JA, Wolpole BG, et al: Munchausen's syndrome: a study of the casualty "black books" of Melbourne. Med J Aust 143:561–563, 1985

Newberger EH: Intervention in child abuse, in Clinical Handbook of Child Psychiatry and the Law. Edited by Schetky DE, Benedek EP. Baltimore, MD, Williams & Wilkins, 1992, pp 145–161

Nichols GR, Davis GJ, Corey TS: In the shadow of the Baron: sudden death due to Munchausen syndrome. Am J Emerg Med 8:216–219, 1990

Rand DC: Munchausen syndrome by proxy as a possible factor when abuse is falsely alleged. Issues in Child Abuse Accusations 1:32–34, 1989

Repper J: Munchausen syndrome by proxy in health care workers. J Adv Nurs 21:299–304, 1995

Sadler JZ: Ethical and management considerations in factitious illness: one and the same. Gen Hosp Psychiatry 9:31–36, 1987

Samuels MP, McClaughlin W, Jacobson PR, et al: Fourteen cases of imposed upper airway obstruction. Arch Dis Child 67:162–170, 1992

Schreier HA, Libow JA: Hurting for Love: Munchausen by Proxy Syndrome. New York, Guilford, 1993

Sigal M, Gelkopf M, Levertof G: Medical and legal aspects of the Munchausen by proxy perpetrator. Med Law 9:739–749, 1990

Sigal M, Altmark D, Gelkopf M: Munchausen syndrome by adult proxy revisited. Isr J Psychiatry Relat Sci 28:33–36, 1991

Sutherland AS, Rodin GM: Factitious disorders in a general hospital setting: clinical features and a review of the literature. Psychosomatics 31:392–399, 1992

World Medical Association: Declaration of Geneva, reprinted in Ethics in Medicine: Historical Perspectives and Contemporary Concerns. Edited by Reiser SJ, Dyck AJ, Curran WL. Cambridge, MA, MIT Press, 1977

Yassa R: Munchausen's syndrome: a successfully treated case. Psychosomatics 19:242–243, 1978

Yorker BC: Nurses accused of murder. Am J Nurs 88:1327–1332, 1988

Yorker BC, Kahan BB: The Munchausen syndrome by proxy variant of child abuse in the family courts. Juvenile and Family Court Journal 42:51–58, 1991

CHAPTER 5

Factitious Disorders and Litigation

Stuart J. Eisendrath, M.D.
Deirdre Conway Rand, Ph.D.
Marc D. Feldman, M.D.

Factitious disorders are well known to any psychiatrist who has worked in a general hospital setting. A patient's willful production of signs and symptoms of disease is one of the most intriguing and publicized conditions found in that setting. For nonpsychiatrists, however, factitious disorders are largely unknown. Lay individuals often have difficulty grasping the concept of factitious disorders. Most people find factitious behavior counterintuitive.

As a result, in the legal setting, factitious disorders cause significant confusion. Those who work within the legal system are accustomed to people who use deception for their own self-interest, such as the criminal who fabricates an alibi or the plaintiff who exaggerates his or her distress for compensation. Police, attorneys, judges, and juries are less familiar with individuals who deceive for the less tangible but equally compelling psychological benefits of playing the patient and/or victim role.

People with factitious disorders produce signs and symptoms of illness for reasons that are not readily explained by external rewards (American Psychiatric Association 1994; Reich and Gottfried 1983). These individuals may engage in serious self-damaging behavior for the apparent sake of assuming the sick role. In this chapter, the authors illustrate ways in which people may transfer this type of pathology from the medical to the legal arena.

Case Reports

Case 1

Ms. A, a 28-year-old medical technologist, was referred for evaluation by her attorney. She was involved in a lawsuit against a pharmaceutical company. Her husband, who was 20 years older than she, had rescued her from a series of physically and sexually abusive relationships. Shortly after he was involved in an accident with serious injuries, Ms. A presented with painful eyes to the local emergency room. Examination revealed severe corneal burns. She claimed they had developed after she had used an over-the-counter eye solution. She was referred to an ophthalmologist for treatment. The ophthalmologist tested the eye solution and determined that lye had been added to it, producing a highly caustic agent. Police investigation revealed no evidence of product tampering prior to the sale of the eye solution.

The corneal injuries healed with treatment consisting of atropine eye drops and patching. Soon, however, Ms. A complained of difficulty with visual acuity. A retinal specialist determined that Ms. A had burned large areas of her retinal surfaces by staring at the sun through binoculars while using the atropine eye drops. She became blind as a result, although her retinas superficially healed and appeared normal on examination. Her husband, not aware of her role in producing the blindness, encouraged her to pursue litigation with the manufacturer of the eye solution. An attorney took her case and filed suit despite having all of her medical records. He referred her to another ophthalmologist without the records. The ophthalmologist found no evidence of physical abnormality on examination and suggested her blindness was a conversion disorder.

She was then referred for psychiatric consultation. The consultant reviewed all of her medical records and realized the factitious nature of her blindness as specified in the retinal specialist's evaluation. The consultant examined Ms. A and learned that she had produced the eye injuries after her husband's accident generated the fear of losing him. In fact, Ms. A stated that she was involved in the lawsuit only at her husband's urging and that she herself had no interest in it. She described how her husband's accident had activated fears of abandonment that Ms. A had experienced in her childhood. There was no evidence of any affective or thought disorder. The psychiatric consultant explained the findings of factitious disorder to her astounded attorney, formulating that her husband's accident had activated feelings that she attempted to resolve by producing the blindness. The attorney withdrew the lawsuit.

Case 2

Ms. B was a 28-year-old woman who was suing a hospital and physician for malpractice and false imprisonment. She had been admitted to a gynecology floor with pelvic pain. Initially, she was treated for presumed pelvic inflammatory disease, but her diagnostic evaluation revealed no evidence of infection. Her gynecologist informed her of this finding and suggested psychiatric referral. She interpreted this suggestion as an accusation that she had no organic problem. She then became enraged at the gynecologist, throwing objects at him in her hospital room. She told a nurse that she had a gun at home and was feeling so depressed that she might use it. A psychiatric consultant assessed her as being at risk for suicide and transferred her involuntarily to a locked psychiatric unit. She became calm rapidly over the next 24 hours and was transferred to a voluntary unit for another 7 days. She was treated primarily for depression and severe marital discord.

The defense attorney asked for psychiatric consultation regarding the case. The attorney furnished medical records extending into the plaintiff's childhood. They disclosed multiple visits to different clinics for various somatic complaints without apparent organic basis. There were also records indicating that she had enjoyed telling tall tales as a child; she had once accused a babysitter of molesting her, but her mother had refused to believe it because of the lack of any evidence. After that, the patient had the persistent belief that she was not being believed in many circumstances, including visits with physicians. During multiple hospitalizations, she developed episodes of fever of unknown origin and was believed to have factitiously elevated her temperature. She had been hospitalized psychiatrically in the past after feigning a suicide attempt "to make sure they admitted me." Her attorney withdrew the case after deposition of the defense expert witness who identified her as having both somatization and factitious disorders.

Case 3

Ms. C was referred for psychiatric evaluation by her attorney. She was the plaintiff in a lawsuit claiming inadequate security by a parking garage company. Her attorney described her as a valiant single mother who had fought many odds to become a successful executive earning $60,000 per year before being mugged in the parking garage. No one witnessed the mugging, but Ms. C described suffering several blows to her head. She had a superficial abrasion on her forehead. After the mugging, Ms. C had a marked loss of intellectual functioning and was no longer able to work at her company. She was involved with a neuropsychologist and psychiatrist in long-term rehabilitation for a postconcussion injury.

The psychiatric consultant received virtually all of Ms. C's medical records extending to childhood. The consultant noted that Ms. C had had several neuropsychological assessments that showed substantial worsening over time since the initial injury. The consultant also reviewed medical records indicating Ms. C had been psychiatrically hospitalized with behavioral problems and possible schizophrenia as an adolescent. During that lengthy hospitalization she was noted to make several false allegations of sexual and/or physical abuse. She eventually recovered and returned home. She then attended college and became a part-time medical laboratory researcher. Following a breakup with a boyfriend, she suffered a fall at work and injured her head. A worker's compensation evaluation at that time found that she had suffered significant organic brain injury and rated her as permanently disabled. After that settlement, she completed 18 months of rehabilitation and returned to college. She graduated from an elite university with highest honors and obtained a master's degree in business administration. She worked successfully in a corporation for 6 years until her alleged mugging.

During examination, the psychiatric consultant learned that the mugging occurred on the day following the end of a long-term relationship with a boyfriend. She interpreted the ending to be a rejection by her boyfriend. She then became highly dependent on her teenage son, who had had to take charge of many household functions she had previously performed. Ms. C's previously active and rewarding social life became restricted to visits to doctors and her rehabilitation program. Mental status examination revealed apparently marked cognitive dysfunction, although some inconsistencies were noted. Imaging studies were completed, including normal magnetic resonance imaging and positron emission tomography scans of the head.

The psychiatric consultant suggested to Ms. C's attorney that her case represented a factitious disorder. The consultant believed there was a conscious component to her presentation as suggested by worsening performance with time on neuropsychological testing. Furthermore, her prior lies about physical and sexual abuse while psychiatrically hospitalized reinforced the impression of a conscious pattern of fabrication. The conscious quality weighed against a diagnosis of conversion disorder. Her prior history of apparent permanent brain injury with complete functional recovery also suggested that a similar coping mechanism was operating this time as well. Although malingering was considered strongly in the differential diagnosis, factitious disorder was given the highest likelihood, since the secondary costs of Ms. C's disorder were extremely high. The disorder appeared to be a reaction to the loss of her romantic relationship and not initiated for financial gain. The gratification of dependency wishes by way of her disorder appeared to be a central factor as well. The psychiatric consultant explained the findings to the plaintiff's attorney, who rapidly settled the case before expert deposition was begun.

Case 4

Ms. D was a seemingly blind woman who was 31 years old when she obtained a restraining order against her brother and cousin. She did this after urging by her therapist, who was alarmed by Ms. D's complaints that her brother and cousin often stopped by her apartment and molested her, sometimes causing bruises or drugging her. Ms. D would bolster her story by showing her therapist bruises on her arm. The judge granted the restraining order. At the hearing, Ms. D's parents told her attorney, "She's made this type of allegation before."

Ms. D had obtained social security disability on the basis of her blindness. She had a seeing eye dog and read braille. Volunteers transcribed books into braille for her. At different points, she appeared for her therapy sessions with her arm in a half cast, claiming that she had tripped, fallen, and fractured her arm. The therapist found these claims surprising, since Ms. D was never noted to stumble or have trouble knowing where she was going despite her blindness. At one point Ms. D indicated that she had developed epilepsy and was taking phenytoin. Shortly after that, the therapist received a call from the neurologist stating that he believed Ms. D was faking epilepsy. On several occasions the therapist had also been told by others that they suspected that Ms. D was not really blind.

Ms. D indicated that periodically her brother and cousin still came by and molested her, though she admitted that she never called the police to enforce the restraining order. Instead, she moved several times to new apartments to "get away from them." They always seemed to find her, nonetheless. It was in the course of trying to effect one of these moves that she came across a landlord who refused to rent to her because of her seeing eye dog. Ms. D retained an attorney and sued the landlord for discrimination against the blind and received a settlement.

After several years in therapy, Ms. D staged an episode that led her therapist to send the police to her house. Ms. D told the police that she and her cousin had struggled, then he raped her, sticking a knife up her vagina. The police took her to the hospital, where she was examined. There was no evidence of rape or any sexual contact, though her blood alcohol level was very high and she appeared distraught. She was held overnight on the psychiatric ward for observation. Her therapist insisted on talking to the police, who indicated that there were no signs of a struggle in Ms. D's apartment. Instead, when they arrived, she was sitting on the couch trying to cut her wrists with a dull pocket knife. The therapist reviewed Ms. D's thick file and realized that Ms. D had never reported molestation to her previous therapists, nor to any of the other doctors and counselors involved in her case. She seemed carefully to select what symptoms she reported to whom. The therapist confronted Ms. D, who denied making up the assaults by the brother and cousin.

The therapist conferred with Ms. D's primary care physician. He felt that the minor elective surgeries Ms. D had convinced another physician to perform were medically unnecessary. He had no record of Ms. D's ever fracturing her wrist or breaking her ribs, though she had asked him for wrapping tape on several occasions. He and the therapist agreed that Ms. D suffered from chronic factitious disorder, including feigned blindness. They decided to confront her gently with everything but her blindness, which seemed necessary to help her organize her existence and stave off a psychotic process. Shortly after that, Ms. D moved to a new city where she was admitted to an inpatient eating disorders program. When the program's staff contacted the previous therapist, they reported that Ms. D had vague memories of being molested as a child, but she was not sure by whom. They were trying to help her recover these memories. The therapist explained that Ms. D suffered from factitious disorder and that she had used factitious rape as a means to get her therapist's attention. The staff person from the eating disorders program had not been familiar with factitious disorders and had thought that the best thing to do was to help Ms. D recover her memories of traumatic rape as a child. After discussion with the therapist, the staff person modified the treatment plan for the patient.

Case 5

Ms. E was a 30-year-old woman who first presented to the police as the traumatized victim of anonymous letters that contained threats of bodily injury and sexual violence to herself and her superior at work. As a result of the letters, Ms. E and her supervisor had a closer relationship. She also began to report receiving anonymous phone calls threatening her, and she promptly informed the police each time a call was received. Once she warned the police that a new threatening letter was going to appear because she had found traces of such a letter on an office typewriter ribbon. Police investigated her suggestion that a disgruntled male co-worker was making the threats. Through fingerprint and typewriter ribbon analysis, they discovered that Ms. E appeared to be writing the letters herself.

After circumstantial evidence mounted to an incontrovertible level, criminal charges were filed against Ms. E. The trial judge ordered Ms. E to undergo psychiatric consultation. She persisted in denying her guilt, even when it emerged that she had been forced to leave her previous job after writing threatening letters to herself and her supervisor. Her history included a claim of sexual assault during adolescence that was determined to be false. She had at least one factitious episode in college, where she injured herself on the head with a hammer and then claimed to have been attacked by an intruder. Another college incident, in which she shoplifted items from the campus bookstore, had resulted in her being dismissed from school. She described several other petty thefts that she had committed in settings where she was likely to be detected.

Ms. E claimed to have been physically and emotionally abused by her father. From early childhood on, Ms. E yearned for her mother to save her from her father, but the passive mother would only defer to him out of fear for herself. Psychiatric examination disclosed no evidence of depression or thought disorder. She denied any dissociative symptoms. Her presumed posttraumatic stress disorder symptoms appeared to lack authenticity. The consultant hypothesized that Ms. E had produced the factitious claim of posttraumatic stress disorder in order to appear to be a victim. This status, in turn, could bring her closer to her female superior, whom she admired, while focusing blame on a male co-worker who symbolically represented her father. After the psychiatric consultant submitted his report to the court, Ms. E's attorney received an anonymous letter pleading for Ms. E not to be sent to jail. Ms. E's attorney had been a staunch believer in her innocence. When he turned this letter over to the police, however, he was outraged to learn that the fingerprints belonged to Ms. E. The consultant advised court-supervised psychotherapy for 3 years with a therapist fully informed of the factitious nature of her disorder. The judge agreed to this condition; because of the distress to her superior and other co-workers, however, he also sentenced her to 6 months of jail.

Discussion

The cases described here illustrate some of the modes in which factitious disorders can penetrate the legal system. Attorneys, judges, and law enforcement personnel are often taken in by such a patient. As with most lay persons, they do not suspect that individuals will do something overtly harmful to themselves. Often, these patients appear to be extremely believable and, in some instances, heroic. This picture is similar to that found in factitious disorder by proxy, where the mothers typically appear "perfect" when others are viewing their behavior (Epstein et al. 1987).

Attorneys representing the patients in the previously mentioned cases uniformly believed in the validity of their clients' statements. In some instances, the attorney's belief may have been bolstered by financial self-interest. For example, in Cases 1 and 3, if the clients' claims were genuine, the damages involved would likely have been greater than 1 million dollars each, with proportionate legal fees. Even when financial considerations are not prominent, as in Cases 4 and 5, there appears to be a propensity for attorneys to believe in their clients' positions. This dynamic similarly applies to the numerous primary physicians who are surprised to discover after many years that their patient has a factitious disorder. In factitious disorder by proxy, some management strategies specifically exclude the pediatrician from the confrontation, because they often refuse to accept that the mother has produced the illness (Waller 1983).

There are several clues to the diagnosis of factitious disorder that emerge from these cases. In some instances, the attorney's staunch belief in his or her client's position is in clear contradiction to the evidence at hand, as in Case 1. Another clue rests with the nature of the act involved. In all of these cases, there was no eyewitness to the injuries or assaults besides the patient/victim. The lack of corroboration by outside witnesses can help suggest the possibility of a factitious disorder, as it did in Cases 1, 3, and 4. In Case 2, there were witnesses, but they did not endorse the plaintiff's claim.

Another important clue to the possibility of a factitious disorder diagnosis is the existence of a psychiatric disorder in the individual's history. All of the individuals were regarded as apparently "normal" by colleagues and attorneys. Nonetheless, all had been in psychiatric treatment at some point in the past, commonly for depressive episodes, behavioral difficulties as adolescents, or suicide attempts. They often appeared to have personality disorders, with borderline, dependent, and antisocial traits, and a paucity of mature defenses. All of the subjects reported that they had been either physically or sexually abused as children, although often the medical record questioned the veracity of these accounts.

At times, however, our subjects seemed to be unconsciously processing traumatic childhood events through their factitious disorders. They may have chosen medical symptoms as a vehicle for interaction with both physicians and attorneys. Getting the interest and support of an attorney, as a symbolic authority figure, may play a role similar to getting the longed-for attention of a neglectful parent. Indeed, these interpersonal issues may have been related to the finding that four of these subjects had some connection with work in the health care field. This vocational choice may allow individuals to act out many of the issues that are prominent in factitious disorders (Folks and Houck 1993). These individuals may select health care occupations so that they may alternately give and receive the care and nurturance that plays a central role in their disorder.

In the cases described previously, the spread of the factitious disorder to the legal setting often occurred secondarily. For example, in Case 1, the litigation took place only at the urging of a spouse. In our litigious society, it is unusual for some form of bodily damage to occur without legal action being strongly considered. If Ms. A had not gone along with her husband's urging for a lawsuit, it would have been difficult for her to explain to him why without revealing the factitious nature of her disorder. Thus, entering the legal arena may sometimes represent an attempt at face saving.

The medical history plays a central role in the detection of factitious disorder. In many instances, there is documentation of past factitious episodes and falsehoods. These findings can clearly buttress the diagnosis. In addition, the medical history often reveals contradictions that suggest a conscious component to the illness production. For example, in Case 1, there was no apparent reason why Ms. A should have suffered retinal injuries in association with corneal burns. In Case 3, Ms. C's recovery from "permanent" organic brain injury to the point where she could obtain a master's degree proved the earlier diagnosis of brain injury to be incorrect. In Case 2, medical records from different institutions were filled with obviously contradictory reports of various illnesses. Case 2 also highlights the difficulty a single clinician with incomplete records would have in making the correct diagnosis. A forensic consultant with access to multiple records, however, was in a unique position to identify the conflicting stories. This point highlights the key role of the psychiatric consultant making the diagnosis and the importance of accessing and reviewing longitudinal medical records. These and other clues that have been used by forensic reviewers in detecting factitious disorders are summarized in Table 5–1.

These cases add to our understanding of abnormal illness behavior, where signs and symptoms are disproportionate to the biomedical disease present. The factitious underpinnings to these legal cases were not identified until they were well into the legal system, and this inadequate recognition is common. One important reason is that the secondary costs of the disorder far outweigh the secondary gain. For example, Ms. A was a successful health professional earning a significant salary at the time she blinded herself. It would be difficult for many lay people to accept the idea that she blinded herself in order to initiate a lawsuit. Indeed, that was not the primary motivation delineated in her psychiatric assessment. Her primary gain, the resolution of psychological issues such as her fear of abandonment, was the fun-

Table 5–1. Potential indicators of factitious disorder on chart review for the forensic consultant

- Signs and symptoms are not controllable—there is continual escalation, or improvement is reliably followed by relapse
- The magnitude of symptoms consistently exceeds objective pathology and/or there is proved exaggeration of symptoms by patient
- Some findings are determined to have been self-induced or at least worsened through self-manipulation
- There is a remarkable number of tests, consultations, and treatment efforts to little or no avail
- The patient is unusually willing to consent to medical/surgical procedures
- The patient disputes test results
- The patient predicts deteriorations, or there are exacerbations shortly before discharge is to occur
- The patient has sought treatment at numerous facilities
- The patient emerges as an inconsistent, selective, or misleading informant, or he or she is resistive to allowing the treatment team access to outside information sources
- There is a history of medical intervention for secondary problems that leads observers to state that the patient must be remarkably unlucky or accident-prone
- Factitious disorder diagnosis is explicitly considered by at least one health care professional
- The patient is noncompliant with diagnostic/treatment recommendations and/or is disruptive on the unit
- The patient focuses on his or her self-perceived "victimization" by the medical and other systems
- There is evidence from laboratory or other tests that disputes information provided by the patient
- The patient has a history of working in the health care field
- The patient engages in gratuitous, self-aggrandizing lying
- While seeking medical/surgical intervention, the patient opposes psychiatric assessment

damental motivation. The litigation was an ancillary development. Case 3 demonstrates a similar set of circumstances. Ms. C did not need to pursue a lawsuit to obtain financial security. The initiating event in her case was the breakup in her relationship; the lawsuit developed initially as a secondary event, although it grew in importance over time. Table 5–2 displays these concepts graphically and demonstrates the differentiation between malingering and factitious disorders. In malingering, the secondary gain (money or relief from a noxious situation) is greater than the secondary costs (loss of income or prestige). This point is illustrated by the observation that malingering patients are rarely willing to induce as much actual bodily injury as factitious disorder patients. With malingering, an outside observer could identify external rewards without knowing anything about the individual's psychological motivations (Binder and Rohling 1996). On the other hand, with factitious disorders, the apparent secondary costs are usually greater than the secondary gain. What ignites the factitious disorder, then, is the primary gain of gratifying a psychological need. The gain for the individual, however, is not usually apparent to an outside observer. The observer would have to hypothesize a psychological motivation for the factitious disorder, since relatively little secondary gain is evident.

In both malingering and factitious disorders, the signs and symptoms of disease are produced consciously. Only factitious disorders have psychological motivations that are usually regarded as unconscious (American Psychiatric Association 1994; Eisendrath 1984). For example, Ms. A did not admit that she blinded herself to receive care or prevent abandonment. Rather, these motivations were inferred by the examiner. In contrast, with malingering, no inference of unconscious process is needed if the situational factors are fully known. Thus, factitious disorders can conceptually be differentiated from malingering by the clarifica-

Table 5–2. Differentiation of malingering and factitious disorders

Malingering:	secondary gain > secondary cost
Factitious disorder:	secondary cost > secondary gain BUT primary gain > secondary cost

tion of whether the motivations are conscious or unconscious (Overholser 1990). Nonetheless, in practice, the demarcation between conscious and unconscious motivations may be difficult to determine at times (Weintraub 1995). For example, as discussed in Chapter 10, "Personal and Interpersonal Toll of Factitious Disorders," some patients have been known to feign or induce illness with the conscious motivation of obtaining nurturance.

The conscious production of symptoms in both malingering and factitious disorders differentiates these conditions from conversion, somatization, and pain disorders, and hypochondriasis (Eisendrath 1984; also see Chapter 2). In the legal setting, there are ways to identify behaviors as consciously produced that are often not available in the general hospital. Exhaustive document review can be revealing. Ms. B's complete medical records gave evidence of her contradictory reports to different physicians. Physical evidence can also be enlightening in cases in the legal setting. For example, fingerprint analysis, DNA analysis, and other forensic techniques have been used to identify cases as being factitious.

The phenomenon of factitious disorders in the legal setting raises some significant heuristic questions. What should we call factitious behavior when it occurs outside of a medical setting? In some instances, obtaining the sick role, the *sine qua non* for the diagnosis of factitious disorders in DSM-IV (American Psychiatric Association 1994), does not really apply. For example, when the primary motivation for the behavior is other than obtaining medical care, such as accruing "victim status," what is the appropriate terminology? DiVasto and Saxton (1992) have reported the case of a police officer who self-inflicted an injury to be accepted by other officers in an elite strike unit, since all the others had experienced attacks. In McDowell's (1987) report, a serviceman disguised his suicide as a murder in the line of duty in order to merit a "hero's" burial. Feldman et al. (1994) and Kanin (1994) have noted that false allegations of rape have been associated with a number of motivations deriving from the victim role. These have included gaining attention and sympathy, seeking revenge, and providing an alibi. Thus, the primary focus of many individuals who feign injury, rape, or illness may be much broader than obtaining the sick role. DSM-IV's category of factitious disorder not otherwise specified might be more useful if broadened by taking into account other intangible goals besides the sick role.

Social commentators have suggested that it was inevitable that factitious presentations would go beyond the medical arena and exploit the response of other social systems. Sinanan and Haughton (1986) observed that "by their very nature, factitious illnesses must be adaptive to changing circumstances, or they would be too obvious. . . . The probable range of variations in the presentation of Munchausen Syndrome is likely to develop in parallel with the evolution of medical and social services." These other services now include mental health clinics and psychiatric hospitals as well as the legal system. As noted in Chapter 3, by the 1980s, frequent reports had begun to appear of patients presenting for psychiatric services with feigned psychosis (Gelenberg 1977; Pope et al. 1982; Popli et al. 1992), falsified bereavement (Phillips et al. 1983; Snowdon et al. 1978), and factitious posttraumatic stress disorder (Resnick 1988; Sparr 1995; Sparr and Pankratz 1983). Observations from the cases that we have described suggest that the extension of factitious behaviors into the legal arena is proceeding apace.

In fact, the cases in this chapter raise the hypothesis that the patient role may be interchangeable with the "aggrieved" or "victim" role for some people. There appears to be a continuum for individuals with factitious behavior; some limit their behavior to the medical arena while others appear primarily to portray a societal "victim" role. Most cases appear to represent a point on the continuum that combines some elements of both the patient and victim roles.

There are significant similarities between the patient and victim roles. Just as patients present themselves to the medical establishment, people who feel aggrieved or victimized present themselves to the legal system. Each system has a well-developed pattern of response to persons who come to them in the defined role. Overall, this consistency enables the systems to respond efficiently and effectively to the large populations they serve. Nonetheless, persons with factitious behaviors may penetrate deeply into the medical or legal system before they are detected. In the medical setting, we know that individuals with factitious disorders have been successful in convincing physicians to perform highly invasive procedures. Similarly, some cases of undiagnosed factitious disorder, many of them similar to the ones presented above, enter the legal system, culminating in a trial and a verdict based on the assumption that the factitious presentation was legitimate. Feldman and Ford (1994) describe several such cases based upon fallacious complaints of medical malpractice.

In one of these cases, a woman's infatuation with her cardiothoracic surgeon led her repeatedly to infect her incision site with feces. In this way she kept him involved continuously in her care. Following the doctor's discovery of the dissimulation and confrontation of the patient, she sued him for negligence, disclaiming involvement in the constant reinfection of the surgical site. Despite compelling evidence that she had infected herself, her "normal" appearance in the courtroom led some jurors to reject the possibility of a psychiatric problem such as factitious disorder, and a hung jury resulted. When the case was retried, the defendant's attorneys deemphasized the diagnosis, speaking instead to the adequacy of his ongoing care of the patient. This time the surgeon was found not liable.

Another malpractice case, *Cohen v. Albert Einstein Medical Center,* also involved a consideration of factitious disorder. Ms. Cohen filed a claim against Albert Einstein Medical Center to recover damages for an injury to her left arm and hand. Briefly, she had been hospitalized in 1982 for arthritis pain, and her physician prescribed meperidine and hydroxyzine by intramuscular injection. An unidentified nurse, according to Ms. Cohen's testimony, administered an injection into her left upper arm; as the injection was being given, Ms. Cohen felt a shock run down her arm into all of her fingers. Her left hand then dropped uselessly at the wrist, and the immobility persisted. Ms. Cohen alleged that her injury was the result of an injection performed negligently. The jury awarded her $1,300,000, though the trial court granted a remittitur to $500,000. Ms. Cohen died of unrelated medical problems in 1989.

Einstein appealed the verdict, and with Ms. Cohen's brother now representing the estate, the appeal was heard in 1991. The appellate court heard arguments that Einstein had intended to prove that Ms. Cohen had Munchausen syndrome and that she had either fabricated her injury or produced it herself. For example, there was never any hospital record indicating that the implicated injection had even been given. However, the trial court had refused to allow the jury to receive this information and had not permitted Einstein's psychiatric expert to testify to it. The appellate court found that the jury had indeed been deprived of information that was relevant to its judgment—namely, the credibility of Ms. Cohen's testimony. It remanded the case for a new trial, and the plaintiffs decided not to proceed further (Janofsky 1994).

Conclusion

Factitious disorders have always been intriguing to physicians, psychiatrists in particular. Psychiatrists and psychologists often have a key role in recognizing such cases in the legal setting. By identifying cases, explaining concepts, and participating in dispositional determinations, these consultants can educate other professionals who may never have heard of a factitious disorder. With increased awareness, the legal community may be better able to contend with the challenges of factitious disorders.

References

American Psychiatric Association: Diagnostic and Statistical Manual of Mental Disorders, 4th Edition. Washington, DC, American Psychiatric Association, 1994, pp 471–475

Binder LM, Rohling ML: Money matters: a meta-analytic review of the effects of financial incentives on recovery after closed-head injury. Am J Psychiatry 153:7–10, 1996

Cohen v Albert Einstein Medical Center, 592 A.2d 720 (Pa. 1991)

DiVasto P, Saxton G: Munchausen's syndrome in law enforcement. FBI Law Enforcement Bulletin 4:11–14, 1992

Eisendrath SJ: Factitious illness: a clarification. Psychosomatics 25:110–117, 1984

Epstein MA, Markowitz RL, Gallo DM, et al: Munchausen syndrome by proxy: considerations in diagnosis and confirmation by video surveillance. Pediatrics 80:220–224, 1987

Feldman MD, Ford CV: Patient or Pretender: Inside the Strange World of Factitious Disorders. New York, Wiley, 1994, pp 193–206

Feldman MD, Ford CV, Stone T: Deceiving others/deceiving oneself: four cases of factitious rape. South Med J 87:736–738, 1994

Folks DG, Houck CA: Somatoform disorders, factitious disorders, and malingering, in Psychiatric Care of the Medical Patient. Edited by Stoudemire A, Fogel B. New York, Oxford University Press, 1993, pp 267–287

Gelenberg AJ: Munchausen's syndrome with a psychiatric presentation. Dis Nerv Syst 38:378–380, 1977

Janofsky JS: The Munchausen syndrome in civil forensic psychiatry. Bull Am Acad Psychiatry Law 22:489–497, 1994

Kanin EJ: False rape allegations. Arch Sex Behav 23:1–6, 1994

McDowell CP: Suicide disguised as murder: a dimension of Munchausen Syndrome. J Forensic Sci 32:254–261, 1987

Overholser JC: Differential diagnosis of malingering and factitious disorder with physical symptoms. Behav Sci Law 8:55–65, 1990

Phillips MR, Ward NG, Ries RK: Factitious mourning: painless patienthood. Am J Psychiatry 140:420–425, 1983

Pope H, Jonas JM, Jones B: Factitious psychosis: phenomenology, family history and long-term outcome of nine patients. Am J Psychiatry 139:1480–1486, 1982

Popli AP, Masand PS, Dewan MJ: Factitious disorders with psychological symptoms. J Clin Psychiatry 53:315–318, 1992

Reich P, Gottfried LA: Factitious disorders in a teaching hospital. Ann Intern Med 99:240–247, 1983

Resnick PJ: Malingering of posttraumatic disorders, in Clinical Assessment of Malingering and Deception. Edited by Rogers R. New York, Guilford, 1988, pp 84–103

Sinanan K, Haughton H: Evolution of variants of the Munchausen syndrome. Br J Psychiatry 148:465–467, 1986

Snowdon J, Solomons R, Druce H: Feigned bereavement: twelve cases. Br J Psychiatry 133:15–19, 1978

Sparr LF: Post-traumatic stress disorder: does it exist? Neurol Clin 13:413–429, 1995

Sparr L, Pankratz LD: Factitious posttraumatic stress disorder. Am J Psychiatry 140: 1016–1019, 1983

Waller DA: Obstacles to the treatment of Munchausen by proxy syndrome. J Am Acad Child Psychiatry 22:80–85, 1983

Weintraub MI: Chronic pain in litigation: what is the relationship? Neurol Clin 13:341–349, 1995

CHAPTER 6

Factitious Disorder by Proxy: Clinical Features, Detection, and Management

Barbara M. Ostfeld, Ph.D.
Marc D. Feldman, M.D.

The fourth edition of the *Diagnostic and Statistical Manual of Mental Disorders* (DSM-IV) defines the essential characteristic of factitious disorder by proxy (FDP) as "the deliberate production or feigning of physical or psychological signs or symptoms in another person who is under the individual's care" (American Psychiatric Association 1994, p. 725). In official psychiatric nomenclature, *factitious disorder by proxy* has replaced the term *Munchausen syndrome by proxy,* which came into broad use after Meadow (1977) identified this phenomenon as a variant of the induction or feigning of disease in oneself.

Because FDP is a form of abuse, typically of children and more rarely of another adult (Sigal et al. 1986; Sinanan and Haughton 1986), the term *perpetrator* is used advisedly to refer to the individual who produces or feigns illnesses in another. In this chapter, the authors focus on FDP as a form of medical abuse; in Chapter 7, the author more centrally considers FDP as a form of emotional abuse.

The perpetrator in FDP may be a parent, babysitter, other relative, or other caregiver. Usually, however, the dyad comprises an infant or child and his or her parent. The victims are typically pre- or early verbal (newborns, infants, or toddlers). At times, however, older children, even adolescents, are involved. For example, in a report by Souid and colleagues (1993), a 13-year-old girl presented with unexplained menorrhagia and hematuria; ultimately, the problems were found to have been caused by warfarin administered by her mother. The mother also drew large amounts of blood and altered laboratory data to cover up her activities. In 98% of the 117 FDP cases reviewed by Rosenberg (1987), the abusive parent was the mother, who typically also seemed loving and concerned. This maternal predominance has been substantiated by Schreier and Libow (1993a), who were able to identify only 11 papers of almost 200 on FDP in which the father was the culpable caregiver.

According to DSM-IV, FDP is a diagnosis that accrues to the abusive parent, not the victim, a decision that has been controversial within the field (Meadow 1995; see also Chapter 4). In this respect, factitious disorder and FDP are often identified in the same individual, usually with the former diagnosis being retrospectively identified in a known FDP perpetrator (Alexander et al. 1990; Meadow 1984; Rosenberg 1987; Samuels and Southall 1992). Conversely, a child victimized by FDP is at increased risk for later development of an independent factitious disorder and for becoming an illness-inducing parent (Feldman and Ford 1994). The overlap between factitious disorder (i.e., self-induction or simulation of illness) and FDP (induction or simulation by proxy) is essentially total in the subset of pregnant individuals who, in victimizing the fetus—perhaps by self-inducing infections of the amniotic fluid—also harm themselves (Goodlin 1985; Porter et al. 1994; Sullivan et al. 1991). Because each disorder is a risk factor for the other, the diagnosis of one may lead to recognition of the other; the mysterious medical crises in a mother's health may suddenly become understandable when her FDP behavior is detected.

FDP carries with it profound risks of short- and long-term harm to the victim as well as the risk of death. The parent falsely reports the child's medical history and/or surreptitiously simulates or induces symptoms, compelling the medical community to respond. In doing so, physicians and other health care professionals who treat these children become the parent's unwitting accomplices. As they search for the elusive diagnosis, they fulfill the parent's pathologic wish for sympathy and attention. Their diagnostic and therapeutic procedures, sometimes invasive, extend hospitalization and engender iatrogenic illnesses. This result then validates and compounds the symptoms the parent has manufactured.

The parent with FDP is often remarkably medically sophisticated and creative in the means by which symptoms are induced or suggested. In her review of published cases, Rosenberg (1987) noted that 27% of the mothers were nurses and thus had formal training and access to medical paraphernalia. To create the illusion of medical abnormalities, they might alter laboratory values or taint urine or blood specimens with bacteria or other contaminants. To create signs and symptoms, they might inject poisons, force-feed emetics or cathartics, irritate the child's skin with abrasive products, or starve and dehydrate their infants. For example, a drop of blood in a specimen of the infant's urine creates the impression of hematuria, sodium contamination of the infant's formula can induce seizures, and brief suffocation of a child attached to a home cardiorespiratory monitor documents the occurrence of infantile apnea.

In Rosenberg's (1987) review, 68 different signs and symptoms were noted. Multiple medical afflictions were present in many cases, and the most common medical signs were bleeding (44%), seizures (42%), central nervous system depression (19%), apnea (15%), diarrhea (11%), vomiting (10%), fever (10%), and rash (9%). Six years later, Schreier and Libow (1993a) expanded this list to include over 100 signs and symptoms. New variants in the methods of simulation or induction, as well as in techniques for detection, continue to be identified. In a recent report, for example, otolaryngologists unmasked an attempt to create the signs of periorificial Crohn's disease (Magnay et al. 1994).

FDP perpetrators tend to behave in characteristic ways. They vigorously pursue medical intervention, changing physicians until the desired medical response is obtained. They may be obsequious yet highly controlling. They gratefully welcome invasive procedures and appear less anxious than the medical staff about their children's unresolving illnesses. They may praise and console physicians who are struggling to treat the perplexing illnesses that fail to respond to traditional therapies. Unlike other parents, they refute any apparent improvement in their child's status and are quick to accuse the physician of failing to recognize the severity of the medical problem. If the physician refuses to escalate the management plan, the perpetrator becomes distressed and is likely to seek care elsewhere. The flight to alternative care is reflected in a study that identified indicators of FDP in 64% of pediatric patients who were discharged against medical advice; the incidence rate in a matched control group was only 8% (Jani et al. 1992).

Unlike malingering, FDP does not stem primarily from the pursuit of external incentives such as insurance settlements or disability payments. Instead, one of the parent's most common goals is to assume the sick role vicariously through the child, with the corresponding mobilization of the interest and support of the medical community. Whereas with opportunistic FDP, the perpetrator may also seek financial rewards (e.g., by soliciting funds for the sick child from charitable organizations), the primary motivation remains the sick role.

Often the perpetrator presents as the "ideal" parent who is inseparable from the hospitalized or convalescing child. He or she is integrally involved in rendering care to the child and develops close relationships with hospital staff. The devotion of the parent misleads the medical and nursing staff, thus delaying or thwarting diagnosis. When the diagnosis of FDP is finally made, an outcome that occurs an average of 14.9 months after the initial presentation (Rosenberg 1987), the hospital staff typically feels angry, betrayed, and less trustful of parents in general (Blix and Brack 1988; Klebes and Fay 1995; Light and Sheridan 1990).

Even when a diagnosis is promptly rendered, however, the child remains vulnerable to misguided beliefs and constraints within the legal system. The courts and the public often respond incredulously to what may be seen as self-serving interpretations of circumstantial data by physicians seeking to protect themselves from malpractice suits (Ostfeld 1995; Samuels et al. 1992). Moreover, a diagnosis that satisfies a medical standard may fail to meet the greater degree of proof required in a criminal action (see Chapter 8). Finally, even where the charges against the parent are upheld, the courts may not recognize how intractable his or her behavior can be (McGuire and Feldman 1989). As a result, the long-term management plan may not adequately protect the child from future abuse (Feldman and Ford 1994).

The human cost of failing to diagnose or sustain a charge of child abuse or to adequately protect victims from further abuse is enormous. Although the mother is not consciously seeking to murder the child, her quest to create the illusion or presence of illness results in an estimated mortality rate of 9% (Rosenberg 1987; Schreier and Libow 1993a). Death occurs for several reasons. First, the parent is not always able to distinguish between a debilitating rather than fatal intervention, and may therefore misjudge the dose of toxin or the duration of airway obstruction needed to produce a symptom rather than a fatality. Second, death may result from the increasingly weakened condition of a repeatedly assaulted infant. Third, much to the distress of the physicians who have attempted to diagnose and treat these "mysterious" illnesses, the child may be further weakened by iatrogenic complications.

For older victimized siblings who have been identified only retrospectively and who thus endured an unchallenged and indeterminate period of exposure, the mortality rate is even higher. Meadow (1990) studied a group of 27 victims of repeated suffocation and determined that 55% of this group's older siblings had died suddenly. It seems reasonable to hypothesize that many of the deceased siblings were victims of FDP.

Although short-term morbidity from FDP is invariable, the incidence and type of long-term morbidity are difficult to assess because of limited follow-up data. Rosenberg (1987) estimated that 8% of FDP victims experienced a protracted period of morbidity. In a recent survey of 54 children who remained in the custody of their mothers, 9% had been the objects of additional fabrications, and nearly 20% of this subset experienced long-term effects such as school absences, impaired concentration, and behavior difficulties stemming from the original as well as subsequent abuse (Bools et al. 1993). Psychological morbidity also includes the development of factitious disorder in adolescence (McGuire and Feldman 1989). Libow (1995) studied 10 adult survivors of FDP and reported that they suffered from persistent insecurity and PTSD symptoms. They also tended to avoid even appropriate medical testing and at times exhibited deficits in reality testing.

Delays or failures in diagnosis have consequences that extend beyond the child and his or her siblings. Rosenberg (1987) determined that in 72% of the cases with symptom simulation (e.g., a fictitious history), 95% of the cases with symptom production, and 84% of the cases with both symptom modes, abuse was being inflicted during the hospitalization itself. Administrators and risk management programs have begun to recognize the potential liability of hospitals in these instances (Melfi 1992). The community also suffers because of the economic burden imposed upon health care resources by unnecessary hospitalizations, extensive use of subspecialists, and multiple and often repeated diagnostic procedures (Ostfeld 1995).

Rosenberg (1987) referred to a "disorder of empathy" (p. 558) among perpetrating mothers. She identified depression, loneliness, and isolation as pervasive themes in those cases for which psychological assessments were available. Schreier and Libow (1993a) have expanded on this theme, referring to perpetrating mothers as narcissistic and psychopathic individuals who offer to their children "a masquerade of mothering that springs from childhood roots that were quietly traumatic" (p. 95). They also suggest that an unsatisfactory relationship with a desired but unavailable father contributes to the development of women who are "forever hungry and doomed to pursue at a distance a bizarrely controlling relationship with a powerful physician" (p. 99). The mother's perception of her infant, "*as person*, means less [to her] . . . than the child as an *object* to be used to manipulate an intensively ambivalent relationship with the physician" (p. 11). Concrete reinforcement for Schreier and Libow's perceptive analysis has been provided through covert videotapes (Samuels 1993; Samuels et al. 1992). In contrast to the devoted and often symbiotic parenting style they reveal in public, these abusing mothers are detached from and unresponsive to their infants when their behavior is unwitnessed.

Several facets of the mother's psychosocial history have been successfully documented by objective data and are considered hallmarks of the perpetrator's profile. For example, many authors observe that when the perpetrator is the mother, the husband is typically a distant and uninvolved figure (e.g., Smith and Killam 1994). However, Schreier and Libow (1993a) note that other markers, such as the mothers' revelations about childhood sexual abuse, are less reliable and may be fabricated. Throughout the process of diagnosis and case management, the mother remains an unreliable source of data (see Chapter 7 for additional information about evaluating the abusive parent).

Although an understanding of the etiology of such aberrant behavior is useful to the therapist, it is important to emphasize that FDP remains a criminal act. As Feldman and Ford (1994) emphasize, as a rule these women are not psychotic and cannot be excused from culpability for this crime against their children:

> We say we can explain some of the behavior on the basis of personality disorders [Bools et al. 1994], but as long as they know right from wrong, we hold them responsible. Most of these patients . . . meet the legal definitions of sanity and responsibility. In a similar way, pedophilia is listed by psychiatrists as a mental disorder, but certainly we proceed with the prosecution of adults who feel driven to abuse children sexually. (p. 161)

The primary responsibility of the medical, legal, and social service systems is to protect the rights of the child.

In the remainder of this chapter, we will further review the profile of the perpetrator and diagnostic markers for FDP. We will identify the challenges to improving the speed and accuracy of diagnosis. Finally, we will discuss the long-term issues in protection of the child.

Factitious Disorder by Proxy: A Representative Case

Sullivan and colleagues (1991) reported the case of an 8-year-old girl whose extensive medical problems and unusually complex management needs evoked suspicion. This case displays the classic features of FDP both in the behavior of the mother and in the clues that led to proper diagnosis. It also illustrates many of the markers and diagnostic tools discussed in the sections that follow.

According to the mother, who served as the informant, the child had undergone repeated hospitalizations and evaluations for recurrent vomiting, apnea, seizures, and diarrhea (four of the most commonly induced symptoms of FDP), as well as hypoglycemia and inability to urinate. She claimed that these symptoms had led to a multitude of diagnoses, including hypoglycemia, cholinergic dysautonomia, intestinal pseudo-obstruction, neurogenic bladder, seizure disorder, central apnea, anemia of chronic disease, recurrent urinary tract infections, and global developmental delay. She described a daily management plan that incorporated sleep apnea monitoring, intermittent daytime and continuous nocturnal bladder catheterization, hyperalimentation, and a medication regimen that included phenobarbital, phenytoin, and epoetin alfa. In addition, the mother reported that the child had to be confined to a wheelchair because of "significant weakness." As is common in FDP cases (Baron et al. 1995), the child's medical care was being rendered in part by pediatric gastroenterologists and other subspecialists.

Sullivan and her colleagues quickly identified several signs suspicious for FDP. Although the patient reportedly had undergone 12 surgical procedures to revise the placement of an indwelling central venous hyperalimentation catheter and had an extensive history of hospitalizations, no documentation of any of the procedures, findings, or diagnoses was available. According to the mother, all records had been lost. The findings from an initial examination by Sullivan's team uncovered a contradiction between the mother's description of a medical sign and the actual findings. The child had a normal gait and demonstrated no evidence of weakness. Calls to several of the patient's previous health care providers revealed that they had been baffled by the continuation of symptoms despite normal studies. In other words, the composite data did not make sense. These outside physicians indicated that invasive therapies had been introduced to relieve symptoms, though their etiology had not been clearly established. These interventions had the unfortunate effects of corroborating the mother's claims of medical acuity and engendering iatrogenic morbidity. A possibility of serial abuse emerged when it was learned that an 11-year-old male sibling had had an extensive history of severe, yet inexplicable, gastroenterologic symptoms that resolved shortly after the birth of the identified patient. Finally, the mother-child relationship was found to be intensely symbiotic:

> Early in the hospitalization, the mother refused to leave her daughter for even a few minutes. She would speak for her child . . . and would not allow the nursing staff to administer catheter care or medications. She brought and used hyperalimentation fluid and medications from her own supply. . . . She

> maintained that only her medications were compatible with the child's hyperalimentation. (p. 113)

A multidisciplinary team that included representatives from the child protection case management team met with the parents and was able to arrange for the child to remain hospitalized as her evaluation continued. Her safety was optimized by denying the mother permission to provide any aspect of her daughter's medical care. A psychiatric evaluation was ordered for the family as well. During the phase of hospitalization that followed this meeting, additional findings consistent with FDP were identified. Significantly, symptoms that began only in the presence of the mother failed to occur in her absence. One of the problems that suddenly resolved through this intervention was apnea; although the mother had reported 20 to 30 significant apneic episodes per night, none was detected when the child was transferred to the intensive care unit for observation and study. The father declined to participate in the psychiatric evaluation and was described as remote. A medical episode from the mother's own history may have been consistent with factitious disorder. Child protection records indicated that FDP had been suspected in the case of the older sibling. The parents had thwarted this investigation by transferring custody of the boy to his grandparents in another state. The mother was well liked by the staff and medically knowledgeable. Her knowledge and style temporarily polarized medical and nursing personnel until sufficient evidence of her manipulative behavior emerged. Most significantly, in the absence of continued findings and symptoms, enteral feedings were slowly resumed, hyperalimentation was eliminated, and bladder catheterization was discontinued. In short, in a protected environment in which maternal access was curtailed, the patient's health and development improved remarkably.

Unfortunately, following the child's discharge to an inpatient psychiatric facility for further treatment of the emotional sequelae of her experience, the parents removed the child against medical advice:

> The child protection team was unable to prevent this despite efforts of several health care providers. Evidence that the parents had directly caused this child's illness was felt to be inconclusive. (p. 114)

The judgment had been made by the authorities that, although there was abundant evidence to support a determination that FDP had occurred, it was circumstantial nonetheless. No episodes of actual symptom induction had been witnessed or recorded, nor were any methods for induction, such as toxins, ever identified. The authors report that the child was later admitted to another medical center where invasive interventions were resumed.

This distressing but all-too-common outcome underscores the challenge faced by medical professionals and child protection workers in meeting the burden of proof required for the removal of the child from the home. If the evidence consists only of such traditional, though compelling, FDP markers as synchrony between the presence of mother and the onset of symptoms, it may be dismissed as circumstantial. For the court to agree to set in motion the dramatic steps required for the child's protection (e.g., separation of the child from the family), a very strong case must be made (Samuels and Southall 1992). The legal issues associated with FDP, including an overview of the rules of evidence, are reviewed in Chapter 8.

The report by Sullivan and colleagues (1991) also demonstrates how delayed a diagnosis of FDP can be even in a case with classic features, including related suspicions about a sibling. The mother's manipulative behavior regarding her son and her successful efforts to thwart her daughter's recovery are indicative of the intractability of the abuse and the vulnerability of the victim.

Making the Case for Factitious Disorder by Proxy

In his introduction to Schreier and Libow's (1993a) text, *Hurting for Love,* Meadow writes, "One of the most lonely and difficult periods of my life was in the early years of defining the syndrome; often my accounts were met with disbelief or ridicule" (p. viii). In the ensuing years, a body of supporting literature has developed, and educational programs have reached the public as well as the professional communities involved in the medical and forensic aspects of the syndrome. Mary Sheridan, Ph.D., a cofounder of the National Association of Apnea Professionals, became concerned about the frequency of suspected FDP cases within apnea programs (Light and Sheridan 1990) and helped establish the Munchausen by Proxy Network to advance professional education. Since then, FDP has been featured on television talk shows, news magazines, and dramas as well as in popular magazines and works of fiction. Review articles have been published in medical, nursing, and social work journals (Mercer and Perdue 1993; Rosenberg 1987; Smith and Killam 1994), and some of the literature is now being directed to hospital administrators (Melfi 1992; Ostfeld 1995). Case studies have appeared in subspecialty journals (e.g., Aideyan and Smith 1995; Magnay et al. 1994) and in numerous foreign journals (e.g., Boros et al. 1995; Oyelami et al. 1994). Thus, a topic once covered in several pages of a child abuse text (Ludwig and Kornberg 1992) has now become the exclusive subject of recent books (Levin and Sheridan 1995; Schreier and Libow 1993a).

Despite these great strides in education and visibility, however, knowledge levels among clinicians are highly variable (Hochhauser and Richardson 1994), adversely affecting the accuracy and timeliness of diagnosis. One survey revealed that the awareness level of family practitioners (even of the more familiar term, *Munchausen syndrome by proxy*) was less than half that of pediatricians (46% vs. 96%) (Ostfeld et al. 1993). In the same survey, social workers were significantly less likely than psychiatrists and psychologists to have heard of the syndrome (42% vs. 89% and 69%, respectively) (Ostfeld and Feldman 1996).

These findings are mirrored in the large differences in the professional literature of each discipline in the availability of articles concerning FDP. For example, the authors conducted a search of the *MEDLINE* and *PsycINFO* computer databases for articles on FDP. The search revealed that physicians are strikingly more likely than psychologists to be exposed to material relating to FDP as they look through their journals (Ostfeld and Feldman 1996).

Schreier and Libow (1993b) surveyed pediatric neurologists and gastroenterologists, subspecialists likely to encounter the type of symptoms created by FDP parents, and discovered that the number of cases diagnosed by each respondent ranged from 0 to 15. They hypothesized that the variance among practitioners outstripped that which would have been accounted for by heterogeneity in the population and suggested that it reflected essential differences in awareness of the disorder. Spuriously low estimates of the prevalence of FDP impede the clinician's sensitivity to and confidence in this diagnosis (Ostfeld 1995).

At least three other factors impede the recognition and diagnosis of FDP (Ostfeld 1995). First, the physician who diagnoses FDP is challenged by the realization that in searching for the cause of the presenting symptoms, he or she may have unwittingly subjected the child to discomfort and risk. Second, while child abuse in any form is stressful for health care professionals to address, FDP may be especially difficult. Typically the perpetrator has been superficially gracious and has developed many sympathetic allies among the staff. As noted in the case of Sullivan and co-workers (1991), colleagues may be polarized in their beliefs and initially unwilling to support the clinician who identifies FDP. Finally, the practitioner must confront the prospect that the unsubstantiated disease processes might be a legitimate but uncommon illness that will go on to be diagnosed by others. All types of child abuse are plagued by the problem of false positives and false negatives (Besharov 1986; Garbarino et al. 1987). For example, in one case, the unusual skin manifestations of dermatomyositis were reported to authorities as indications of possible FDP; after recognition of the actual medical diagnosis, a malpractice action by the parents ensued, though the pediatrician's duty to report his suspicions was upheld (Feldman and Allen 1996). In another case, circumstantial evidence was used to convict a mother of murdering her child by antifreeze poisoning. She spent 5 years in prison before it was discovered that her child had died of an unusual disease, one that was little known to the medical community at the time she brought her child for treatment (Schreier and Libow 1993a). As with all accusations of child abuse, the motivations of the accuser should be taken into consideration, including physician attitudes such as overzealousness or anger at discovering that he or she has been misled (D. Rand, personal communication, December 1994). Clear markers, compelling evidence, and a supportive group of colleagues are needed to overcome these stressors (Ostfeld 1995; Stevenson and Alexander 1990).

Similar inhibitions affect other professions involved in the disposition of an FDP case. Judges, attorneys, and police are initially incredulous (Feldman 1994; Samuels and Southall 1992) and must be educated in order to respond helpfully to the needs of the victim. Schreier and Libow (1993a) emphasize the responsibility of the team members involved to provide the courts with appropriate literature. Ideally, physicians and hospital administrators should meet with child protective service agents and representatives of the court proactively to develop a comprehensive program of intervention.

Warning Signs of Factitious Disorder by Proxy

As illustrated previously in the case of the 8-year-old girl with multiple medical problems, there are a number of red flags that should raise the clinician's suspicion that some or all of the signs and symptoms have been fabricated or induced. The list of warning signs in Table 6–1 is based in part on the observations of Feldman and Ford (1994), Guandolo (1985), Meadow (1982), Rosenberg (1987), Samuels and Southall (1992), Schreier and Libow (1993a), Folks (1995), and Sullivan et al. (1991).

The FDP markers in Table 6–1 do not in themselves constitute proof. The diagnosis generally is deduced by examining a broad range of clinical factors, and it does not depend upon the absolute number of warning signs identified in a given case. In a similar way, the items in the list are not necessarily to be weighted equally; for example, the unexplained death of another child in the same family is obviously a more powerful indicator of possible FDP than is an uninvolved and unavailable father. Finally, the absence of many, or even most, of the items in Table 6–1 does not rule out FDP. Instead, once FDP is considered, the physician or other health care professional should meet with the other clinicians who are treating the patient to share information and voice concerns. FDP should be included in the differential diagnosis, and steps should be taken to confirm or eliminate suspicions.

Confirming Suspicions

Once suspicions are raised, a difficult decision must be made. When should confrontation occur? If the parent is approached before suspicions are sufficiently validated, he or she may withdraw the child from the hospital and flee, leaving the physician with too little data upon which protective service and legal

Table 6–1. Warning signs of factitious disorder by proxy

- The symptoms and pattern of illness are extremely unusual, or inexplicable physiologically
- Repeated hospitalizations and work-ups by numerous caregivers fail to reveal a conclusive diagnosis or etiology
- Physiologic parameters are consistent with induced illness (e.g., apnea monitor tracings disclose massive muscle artifact prior to respiratory arrest, suggesting that the child has been struggling against an obstruction to the airways)
- The patient fails to respond to appropriate treatments
- The vitality of the patient is inconsistent with the laboratory findings
- The signs and symptoms disappear when the mother has not had access to the child
- The mother appears less concerned than the clinicians about their inability to identify the cause of the illness
- The mother thrives in the hospital and becomes unusually close to staff
- The mother refuses to go home and insists on caring for the patient herself, perhaps even bringing her own food and medication for the child
- The mother is the only witness to the onset of seizures, apnea, or other signs and symptoms
- The father is rarely encountered
- Either the mother or her other children have had unexplained illnesses
- The mother has had medical or nursing education
- The mother has had exposure to "models" of the illnesses afflicting the child (e.g., a parent with sleep apnea)
- The mother describes catastrophes that have befallen the family during the hospitalization
- The mother welcomes even invasive and painful tests involving the child
- The mother grows anxious if the child improves
- The mother grows defensive if the information she provides is questioned or maternal lying is proved
- Medical records from other hospitals are reported by the mother to be missing, and no other informant is made available
- Medical observations yield information that is inconsistent with parental reports

authorities can build a case. Moreover, if an investigation is launched, the mother or father, once alerted, can temporarily curtail the abuse. On the other hand, if the verification period is extended so that adequate data can be gathered, it is at the expense of the child, who continues to be compromised by the abuse. To a certain extent, the physician's flexibility is limited by each state's mandatory reporting laws for abuse (American Medical Association 1992). At some point, the evidence grows stronger and the child protective service agencies must be notified. Parental notification must follow within 24 hours, once again affecting the physician's ability to gather adequate documentation.

Physicians need the support of a knowledgeable multidisciplinary team in order to address a number of central questions. Team building should begin long before any case is presented, and, to the extent possible, the members should include psychiatrists, other physicians, psychologists, social workers, nurses, law enforcement agents, risk managers, hospital administrators, attorneys, child protection service agents, and court representatives (Siebel et al. 1993). The initial purpose should be to share information about FDP. With insight into its morbidity and mortality rates and the dilemmas faced in gathering evidence, the participants can develop a cooperative plan of action to serve the best interests of the child. For example, a functioning team can determine what degree of concern must exist before protective services agencies are notified, what forensic requirements must be met in order to prosecute a case, what amount of delay the child protective service worker may legally provide before the family must be confronted, and what ethical and legal dilemmas may be posed by employing covert video surveillance.

Covert video surveillance is one of the most effective but controversial methods of gathering objective evidence (Byard and Burnell 1994; Epstein et al. 1987; Ostfeld 1995); in some instances, it provides the only documentation that will establish the case against the parent. The issue of covert video surveillance is discussed more fully in Chapter 8, "Legal Issues in Factitious Disorder by Proxy."

Feldman and Ford (1994), Leonard and Farrell (1992), Mercer and Perdue (1993), Ostfeld (1995), Rosenberg (1987), Samuels and Southall (1992), Schreier and Libow (1993a), and Smith and Killam (1994) have all proposed methods for confirming suspicions.

A summary of their recommendations, some of which may be proscribed at times by legal constraints, is presented in Table 6–2.

If the early suspicions of the team are reinforced and have justified the involvement of child protective services, confrontation of the parents must take place. Authors differ on whether both parents should be present or the mother confronted by herself (Feldman 1994). Regardless, FDP mothers are at risk for becoming suicidal (Rosenberg 1987) and need to be addressed supportively. The focus should be on offering assistance to resolve the crisis. A mental health practitioner should be present or at least immediately accessible, and evaluation should commence at once. To prevent the parent from fleeing with the child, a hold order should be obtained in advance of the meeting. Custody arrangements should be coordinated by the child protection service agent.

Differential Diagnosis

Several categories of illness presentation can be confused with FDP, and care must be taken to distinguish among them. First, overanxious parents may continually bring their children to the office and emergency room, therefore putting their children at risk for overtreatment or complications due to factors such as unnecessary dietary restrictions (Roesler et al. 1994; Pugliese et al. 1987). However, they differ from FDP parents in motivation and reaction. Their efforts to engage physicians are based on a genuine belief that their children are ill and that the physician has overlooked important abnormalities. Typically, both parents are involved in such cases, and, unlike FDP parents, they are relieved when illness is ruled out. The illnesses are usually not exotic, and they respond predictably to medical intervention.

Second, parents of children who are recovering from a documented health crisis such as prematurity may appear to be overprotective and excessive in their reaction to mild symptoms of illness. Levels of responsiveness that were reinforced as appropriate during a severe illness appear excessive once the child's health improves. Such parental behavior is understood when it is placed in the context of their recent experiences. The physician can distinguish these families from abusive ones by documenting

Table 6–2. Recommendations for confirming factitious disorder by proxy

- Convene a multidisciplinary team to discuss suspicions and assist in gathering information, protecting the child, alerting protective service agents, and confronting the parents
- Safeguard the child by restricting visitation and monitoring all encounters with the parent; a court order may be necessary if the parent does not voluntarily comply with restricted visitation
- Obtain toxicologic studies; freeze and store all biologic samples until a plan for analyzing them has been developed; match the child's blood type to that in urine or other samples if signs involving bleeding have been noted; note timing of all laboratory studies, symptoms, and visitation in order to develop a time line of events; analyze nutritional and other supplies brought in by the mother
- Obtain all medical records of the patient, siblings, and parents to verify histories given by the mother; interview as many clinicians as possible from past hospitalizations
- Because confidentiality laws may prohibit the release of such records, the team should determine in advance of any case what restrictions exist and what must be done to obtain records
- Interview relatives to obtain additional independent corroboration of pertinent information provided by the mother
- Safeguard all specimens and medical records so that the mother will not have access to them
- Interview staff to determine the frequency with which episodes originated when the mother and child were alone; note any episodes that originated in the presence of the medical staff while the mother was absent
- Document all findings. Be aware that occasional positive findings on tests or examinations may not be clinically meaningful or explanatory; instead, positive results of debatable significance are likely whenever extensive, repeated testing is performed
- Allow only nursing staff to administer food and medication
- If apnea, cardiac or respiratory arrest, seizures, or loss of consciousness have been reported, set up continuous multichannel physiological recordings to determine the veracity of the reports
- Search the room for poisons, drugs, syringes, and other paraphernalia
- If he or she is verbal, interview the child separately from the mother
- Consider covert video surveillance

the veracity of the previous diagnoses. Once recovery is well established, these parents will begin to attenuate their reactions to illness.

Third, some parents discontinue prescribed medications because of concerns about side effects, not because they wish to mislead medical caregivers. In doing so, they may inadvertently produce the very outcome they had sought to avoid—worsening symptoms. It is possible to elicit their concerns and provide appropriate education and assurance. Unlike the FDP parent, these parents comply after they receive additional information, or at least become more forthright in expressing their reservations about the medication regimen.

Fourth, a parent's deliberate exaggeration of the child's symptoms is not necessarily indicative of FDP, although certainly it too can lead to overtreatment. Unlike the FDP parent who fabricates a history, the parent who exaggerates may be attempting to call attention to symptoms that concern her or him but do not impress the physician. For example, the child's fever may be cited as being higher by a point, or one episode of vomiting may become two. The goal of such untruths appears to be to attract the physician's attention and obtain care. It has been the authors' clinical impression that these parents welcome recovery when it ensues.

Fifth, a number of illnesses present with such variability that it is possible for the same patient to appear remarkably different within a short period of time. An innocent parent may appear to be an illness exaggerator if she or he is describing a child whose symptoms no longer fit his or her description. Asthma falls into this category. If the physician is suspicious that the description of severity is being orchestrated by the parent, it is important to obtain independent corroboration.

Sixth, an older child may malinger for secondary gain. The innocent parent witnesses and presents the child's symptoms to the physician, ultimately appearing to be an illness exaggerator when the report is disconfirmed by the examination.

Finally, a legitimate medical disorder occasionally is presented with symptoms that can be confused with various manifestations of FDP or with child abuse in general. Some of these disorders or syndromes are so rare that the clinician may fail to consider them or may view the possibility as too obscure. Osteogenesis imperfecta, a genetic disorder that results in frequent fractures, fits into this category. Once the diagnosis is entertained, however, it is relatively simple to distinguish from abuse. Other disorders or syndromes are more common and plausible but lack pathognomonic findings that definitively establish the etiology of the symptom. Sudden infant death syndrome (SIDS), the leading cause of death of infants from 1 month to 1 year of age, falls into this category. SIDS is the sudden death of a seemingly healthy infant. Although many promising hypotheses about the underlying causes are currently under study (Howat et al. 1994), the diagnosis is essentially one of exclusion. Therefore, even though SIDS is a well-described phenomenon that is significantly more common than infanticide, the absence of a clear cut marker renders parents vulnerable to charges of abuse. On rare occasions, such charges have been sustained, and the resultant publicity creates additional distress for legitimately bereaved parents. Mindful of their suffering, the Committee on Child Abuse and Neglect of the American Academy of Pediatrics (1994) has endorsed guidelines that will enhance the recognition of infanticide without stigmatizing SIDS families.

Though there are well-publicized exceptions (Associated Press 1990), the prototypical FDP parent seeks to create illness but not to kill. However, suffocation-induced apnea may result in death because parents are not always able to calculate what would constitute a "benign" exposure to asphyxia. Meadow (1990) has observed that frequent bouts of apnea prior to death occur in only 10% of SIDS cases but in up to 90% of children who have been actively suffocated. Such atypical presentations may provide a useful clue in the differential diagnosis. However, it would be an egregious wrong to replace a SIDS diagnosis with one of FDP without objective data. Such differential diagnoses are difficult medically and emotionally, and each case requires careful investigation.

Long-Term Management Plan

The primary goal of any long-term management plan must be the protection of the child. The data strongly underscore the continued vulnerability of children who remain with their parents after a diagnosis is established and children's protective services are involved (Bools et al. 1993; McGuire and Feldman 1989). Moreover, reports of the efficacy of therapeutic interventions with the abusive parent remain discouraging, particularly in cases in which the parent persistently denies culpability (Feldman 1994). Therefore, in most situations, the child's safety can be ensured only by removing him or her from the home. Reunification of families should be undertaken only if the child's continued safety can be guaranteed.

A second goal of management is treatment. For the victimized child, additional medical care to address residual physical problems may be necessary. The child should also receive a psychological-psychiatric evaluation and therapy. Despite the abuse, children remain attached to their parents and suffer from the separation. If possible, perpetrating mothers and other family members should be engaged in long-term therapy. Though, as noted, denial remains a major obstacle to progress, some nonconfrontational interventions have been successfully employed for patients with factitious physical disorders and may be effective for the FDP parent as well (Eisendrath 1989; Griffith and Slovik 1989).

Many researchers and clinicians have offered guidelines for the development of management plans (Feldman 1994; Rosenberg 1987; Samuels and Southall 1992; Schreier and Libow 1993a). Their suggestions form the basis for the recommendations in Table 6–3. Some redundancy in elements of the plan will be evident. However, in light of the mother's ability to manipulate professionals and perpetrate the abuse even in ostensibly protected environments, such vigilance is prudent. These recommendations are more likely to be implemented and enforced if they have been ordered by the court following successful prosecution. Since there is a high rate of recividism, monitoring should be established for an extended period and should continue even if reunification is eventually permitted.

Reunification of the Family

McGuire and Feldman (1989) and Neale et al. (1991) have raised serious concerns about the prospects for a safe reunification, particularly in more severe cases. Actively perpetrating mothers are extremely skillful in convincing case workers and physicians of their innocence. Even therapists who treat the convicted mothers are vulnerable to their influence (Schreier and Libow 1993a). The

Table 6–3. Management recommendations following recognition of factitious disorder by proxy

- The child should be removed from the care of the mother and placed in a custodial situation that will ensure his or her safety. Placement with relatives may not guarantee adequate protection. This separation should continue at least until the mother's evaluation is completed and the child's health status is clarified
- A pediatrician or family practitioner familiar with the case and knowledgeable about FDP should become the long-term, court-ordered gatekeeper for the child's health care needs. He or she should coordinate whatever additional care is required and remain involved with the child
- The gatekeeper should perform a periodic audit of the child's health and school records. The latter may reveal absences or developmental and behavioral disabilities that are associated with FDP
- Given the vulnerability of siblings who may have remained in the custody of the mother, as well as those born subsequently, audits of their health status should be performed for an extended period
- Long-term psychotherapy for both the parents and the child should be provided by clinicians familiar with the disorder
- The mother's interactions with the child should be evaluated because her aberrant parenting may extend into areas other than symptom induction. Any identified deficiencies should be addressed in the treatment plan
- If the family is reunited, supervision should be continued and arrangements made with the courts to have monitoring continue following any relocations
- No distinction should be made between the disease-simulating and the disease-inducing parent. Each is capable of the other form of FDP

Note. FDP = factitious disorder by proxy.

susceptibility of therapists is of critical concern because they must assist the court in making recommendations about a reunion. Schreier and Libow (1993a) comment:

> Rendering responsible mental health consultation on such serious and permanent matters as termination of parental rights is particularly difficult because courts prefer to decide in 6 months or a maximum of 18 months about permanent reunification or separation of a child and his or her parent, thereby increasing pressure on therapists to make very difficult judgments. A therapist treating a mother is susceptible to the patient's dynamics and convincing denials and protestations. We have usually found that the child's therapist, though also susceptible . . . can offer a more objective view of the best interests of the child. . . . (p. 217)

Without objective markers of improvement, the therapist must rely on his or her impressions of the parent's degree of insight and judgment. However, the risks are too great to allow these predictions to serve as principal determinants. Meadow's (1985) and Schreier and Libow's (1993a) thorough reviews of contraindications and stipulations should also be consulted when a reunification plan is being considered. Meadow (1985) suggested that the following situations were indicators of risk for the child who remained in the custody of the mother: a history of severe abuse; abuse during infancy; unexplained deaths of siblings; lack of insight by the mother; manifestations of factitious disorder by the mother; other significant lifestyle risk factors; and persistence of FDP even after discovery. Schreier and Libow (1993a) add other standards that should be met: the parent's partner, spouse, or other relatives should acknowledge what has happened and express the strong desire to protect the child; the mother's therapist should approve of reunification and also provide assurance that no other serious maternal psychopathology has emerged during evaluation or treatment; the parent should demonstrate appropriate parenting skills, including spontaneous displays of empathy; the parent should no longer claim that the child has disorders that have no medical basis; and the child should be free of any substantiated serious medical problems, because the situation would then be fraught with opportunity for the parent to influence physicians anew (Schreier and Libow 1993a).

Conclusion

As the diagnostic indicators become more sensitive and the diagnostic process refined, milder forms of FDP may be detected. It is possible that subtler, less lethal levels may stem from different psychodynamic issues that will be more responsive to treatment. If there is, in fact, a variance in prognosis for the parent based on the severity of the fabrications and illness inductions, then modifications in the management and reunification plans will need to be made. This question remains in need of study. To date, the research that is available on morbidity and mortality, efficacy of therapeutic interventions, and recidivism has tended to involve severe cases, and it has yielded pessimistic findings. We cannot ignore these data.

References

Aideyan UO, Smith WL: Radiological features in a case of Munchausen syndrome by proxy. Pediatr Radiol 25:70–71, 1995

Alexander R, Smith W, Stevenson R: Serial Munchausen by proxy. Pediatrics 86:581–585, 1990

American Medical Association: AMA Medicolegal Guidelines Concerning Child Abuse and Neglect. Chicago, IL, American Medical Association, 1992

American Psychiatric Association: Diagnostic and Statistical Manual of Mental Disorders, 4th Edition. Washington, DC, American Psychiatric Association, 1994

Associated Press: Grief-stricken mother suspected in 7 deaths; deadly pattern repeated time after time since '76. Houston Post, December 27, 1990, p A18

Baron HI, Beck DC, Vargas JH, et al: Overinterpretation of gastroduodenal motility studies: two cases involving Munchausen syndrome by proxy. J Pediatr 126:397–400, 1995

Besharov DJ: Unfounded accusations: a new child abuse problem. The Public Interest 83:18–33, 1986

Blix S, Brack G: The effects of a suspected case of Munchausen's syndrome by proxy on a pediatric nursing staff. Gen Hosp Psychiatry 10:402–409, 1988

Bools C, Neale B, Meadow R: Co-morbidity associated with fabricated illness (Munchausen syndrome by proxy). Arch Dis Child 67:77–79, 1992

Bools CN, Neale BA, Meadow SR: Follow up of victims of fabricated illness (Munchausen syndrome by proxy). Arch Dis Child 69:625–630, 1993

Bools C, Neale B, Meadow R: Munchausen syndrome by proxy: a study of psychopathology. Child Abuse Negl 18:773–788, 1994

Boros SJ, Ophoven JP, Anderson R, et al: Munchausen syndrome by proxy: a profile for medical child abuse. Aust Fam Physician 24:768–769, 772–773, 1995

Byard RW, Burnell RH: Covert video surveillance in Munchausen syndrome by proxy. Med J Aust 160:352–56, 1994

Committee on Child Abuse and Neglect, American Academy of Pediatrics: Distinguishing sudden infant death syndrome from child abuse fatalities. Pediatrics 94:124–126, 1994

Eisendrath SJ: Factitious physical disorders: treatment without confrontation. Psychosomatics 30:383–387, 1989

Epstein MA, Markowitz RL, Gallo DM, et al: Munchausen syndrome by proxy: considerations in diagnosis and confirmation by video surveillance. Pediatrics 80:220–224, 1987

Feldman MD: Denial in Munchausen syndrome by proxy: the consulting psychiatrist's dilemma. Int J Psychiatry Med 24:121–128, 1994

Feldman MD, Allen DB: "False positive" factitious disorder by proxy. South Med J 89:452–453, 1996

Feldman MD, Ford CV: Patient or Pretender: Inside the Strange World of Factitious Disorders. New York, Wiley, 1994, pp 146–169

Folks DG: Munchausen's syndrome and other factitious disorders. Neurol Clin 13:267–281, 1995

Garbarino J, Guttmann E, Seeley JW: The Psychologically Battered Child: Strategies for Identification, Assessment and Intervention. San Francisco, CA, Jossey-Bass, 1987

Goodlin RC: Pregnant females with Munchausen syndrome. Am J Obstet Gynecol 153:207–210, 1985

Griffith JL, Slovik LS: Munchausen syndrome by proxy and sleep disorders medicine. Sleep 12:178–183, 1989

Guandolo VL: Munchausen syndrome by proxy: an outpatient challenge. Pediatrics 75:526–530, 1985

Hochhauser KG, Richardson RA: Munchausen syndrome by proxy: an exploratory study of pediatric nurses' knowledge and involvement. J Pediatr Nurs 9:313–320, 1994

Howat WJ, Moore IE, Judd M, et al: Pulmonary immunopathology of sudden infant death syndrome. Lancet 343:1390–1392, 1994

Jani S, White M, Rosenberg LA, et al: Munchausen syndrome by proxy. Int J Psychiatry Med 22:343–349, 1992

Klebes C, Fay S: Munchausen syndrome by proxy: a review, case study, and nursing implications. J Pediatr Nurs 10:93–98, 1995

Leonard KF, Farrell PA: Munchausen syndrome by proxy: a little-known type of abuse. Postgrad Med 91:197–204, 1992

Levin AV, Sheridan MS (eds): Munchausen Syndrome by Proxy: Issues in Diagnosis and Treatment. New York, Lexington, 1995

Libow JA: Munchausen by proxy victims in adulthood: a first look. Child Abuse Negl 19:1131–1142, 1995

Light MJ, Sheridan MS: Munchausen syndrome by proxy and apnea (MBPA). Clin Pediatr 29:162–168, 1990

Ludwig S, Kornberg AE (eds): Child Abuse: A Medical Reference (2nd Edition). New York, Churchill Livingstone, 1992.

Magnay AR, Debelle G, Proops DW, et al: Munchausen syndrome by proxy unmasked by nasal signs. J Laryngol Otol 108:336–338, 1994

McGuire TL, Feldman KW: Psychologic morbidity of children subjected to Munchausen syndrome by proxy. Pediatrics 83:289– 292, 1989

Meadow R: Munchausen syndrome by proxy: the hinterland of child abuse. Lancet 2:343–345, 1977

Meadow R: Munchausen syndrome by proxy. Arch Dis Child 57:92–98, 1982

Meadow R: Factitious illness: the hinterlands of child abuse, in Recent Advances in Pediatrics. Edited by Meadow R. Edinburgh, Scotland, Churchill Livingstone, 1984

Meadow R: Management of Munchausen syndrome by proxy. Arch Dis Child 60:385–393, 1985

Meadow R: Suffocation, recurrent apnea, and sudden infant death. J Pediatr 117:351–357, 1990

Meadow R: What is, and what is not, "Munchausen syndrome by proxy?" Arch Dis Child 72:534–538, 1995

Melfi MH: Munchausen syndrome by proxy: "please protect me from my parents." Paper presented at the 14th annual conference of the American Society for Healthcare Risk Management, Las Vegas, NV, November 1992

Mercer SO, Perdue JD: Munchausen syndrome by proxy: social work's role. Soc Work 38:74–81, 1993

Neale B, Bools C, Meadow R: Problems in the assessment and management of Munchausen syndrome by proxy abuse. Children and Society 5:324–333, 1991

Ostfeld B: The role of the hospital administration in the diagnosis of Munchausen syndrome by proxy, in Munchausen Syndrome by Proxy: Issues in Diagnosis and Treatment. Edited by Levin AV, Sheridan MS. New York, Lexington, 1995, pp 355–367

Ostfeld BM, Feldman MD: Factitious disorder by proxy: awareness among mental health practitioners. Gen Hosp Psychiatry 18:113–116, 1996

Ostfeld B, Feldman M, Hiatt M, et al: Physician awareness of Munchausen syndrome by proxy. Pediatr Res 30:120A, 1993

Oyelami OA, Alhaj AM, Airede IK: Munchausen syndrome by proxy: a case report and review of the literature. Cent Afr J Med 40: 222–226, 1994

Porter GE, Heitsch GM, Miller MD: Munchausen syndrome by proxy: unusual manifestations and disturbing sequelae. Child Abuse Negl 18:789–794, 1994

Pugliese MT, Weyman-Daum M, Moses N, et al: Parental health beliefs as a cause of nonorganic failure to thrive. Pediatrics 80:175–182, 1987

Roesler TA, Barry PC, Bock SA: Factitious food allergy and failure to thrive. Arch Pediatr Adolesc Med 148:1150–1155, 1994

Rosenberg DA: Web of deceit: a literature review of Munchausen syndrome by proxy. Child Abuse Negl 11:547–563, 1987

Samuels M: ALTEs and Munchausen syndrome by proxy. Presented at the eleventh annual Conference on Apnea in Infancy of the National Association of Apnea Professionals. Rancho Mirage, CA, January 1993

Samuels MP, Southall DP: Munchausen syndrome by proxy. Br J Hosp Med 47:759–762, 1992

Samuels MP, McClaughlin W, Jacobson RR, et al: Fourteen cases of imposed upper airway obstruction. Arch Dis Child 67:162–170, 1992

Schreier HA, Libow JA: Hurting for Love: Munchausen by Proxy Syndrome. New York, Guilford, 1993a

Schreier HA, Libow JA: Munchausen syndrome by proxy: diagnosis and prevalence. Am J Orthopsychiatry 63:318–321, 1993b

Siebel M, Whelan-Williams S, Baker T: Munchausen syndrome by proxy: a hospital's challenge. Paper presented at Fourth European Conference on Child Abuse and Neglect, Padua, Italy, April 1993

Sigal MD, Altmark D, Carmel I: Munchausen syndrome by adult proxy: a perpetrator abusing two adults. J Nerv Ment Dis 174:696–698, 1986

Sinanan K, Haughton H: Evolution of variants of the Munchausen syndrome. Br J Psychiatry 148:465–467, 1986

Smith K, Killam P: Munchausen syndrome by proxy. MCN Am J Matern Child Nurs 19:214–221, 1994

Souid AK, Korins K, Keith D, et al: Unexplained menorrhagia and hematuria: a case report of MBP. Pediatr Hematol Oncol 10:245–248, 1993

Stevenson RD, Alexander R: Munchausen syndrome by proxy presenting as a developmental disability. J Dev Behav Pediatr 11:262–264, 1990

Sullivan CA, Francis GL, Bain MW, et al: Munchausen syndrome by proxy: 1990. A portent for problems? Clin Pediatr 30:112–116, 1991

CHAPTER 7

Comprehensive Psychosocial Assessment in Factitious Disorder by Proxy

Deirdre Conway Rand, Ph.D.

In this chapter, the author discusses the psychosocial assessment issues that arise after factitious disorder by proxy (FDP) has been detected and reported. These issues include determining the appropriate level of intervention and whether the child should be removed from the abusing parent, either immediately or in the long term. In recent years, FDP has been conceptualized as a complex form of emotional abuse that sometimes involves serious physical abuse (Meadow 1991; Neale et al. 1991). This formulation is consistent with prevailing views of psychological maltreatment as the core issue in the broader picture of physical abuse, neglect, and sexual abuse of children (Garbarino et al. 1987).

The clinical picture in FDP may consist of emotional abuse alone, as when the mother's stories of false illness prevent the child from leading a normal life. Although not life threatening, emotional abuse can be severe, causing profound disturbances in the child's psychological and social development. When physical abuse occurs in FDP, for example when a mother (the usual offender) smothers her child to induce seizures, closer examination of the mother-child relationship will reveal the elements of psychological maltreatment that make it possible for the mother willfully to threaten her child's life.

Nowhere is the complex nature of the emotional abuse more apparent than in a contemporary variation of FDP in which the mother presents her child in the victim role, falsely alleging that the child was physically or sexually abused by someone else (Rand 1989, 1990, 1993). At the mother's insistence, the child undergoes repeated physical exams and interviews by police, social workers, and therapists. Meadow (1993a) reports a group of FDP cases in which investigation of the apparently factitious abuse led to the discovery that the mother was simultaneously fabricating illness in her child.

Increased awareness of FDP is likely to result in more reports of emotional abuse alone and of relatively mild or borderline cases. Psychological maltreatment provides a model for evaluating the seriousness of these reports. This model is one of comprehensive assessment that integrates evaluation of the parent, the child, their interaction with one another and with medical personnel, and their larger social context.

Psychological maltreatment refers to patterns of psychologically destructive behavior, such as regular attacks on the child's development of self and social competence. The clinical picture may include emotional neglect, defined as failure to nourish the child's character and self in important ways. Garbarino and colleagues (1987) describe five types of emotional abuse and neglect that are listed below with specific examples involving FDP:

1. **Isolating.** The adult removes the child from normal social experiences, preventing the child from developing friendships and making the child believe that he or she is alone in the world. An FDP mother who regularly keeps her child home from school based on false stories of the child's being ill is isolating her child from normal social and educational experiences. Isolation may also occur when the mother keeps the child psychologically fused with her so that the child has no contact with the external world that is not mediated by the mother.
2. **Terrorizing.** The adult bullies the child or mounts a campaign of verbal or physical attack that makes the child believe that the world is capricious and hostile. In FDP, the child may

be terrorized by the life-threatening crises the mother creates, although unaware that the mother is causing them. A form of terrorizing occurs when the mother barrages her child in placement with so many letters and phone calls that the child's security is disrupted.

3. **Rejecting.** The parent abandons the child physically and/or psychologically, or rejects the child's legitimate physical and emotional needs. In FDP, this term may apply to the young child's experience during long stays in the impersonal hospital environment. Rejection of the child was acted out by a group of mothers who poisoned their children with salt. The mothers on follow-up reported feelings of violence and hatred toward their infants at the time of the poisonings (Meadow 1993b).
4. **Ignoring.** More passive and neglectful than rejecting, ignoring refers to a parent who deprives the child of essential stimulation and responsiveness by virtue of parental incapacity and/or self-preoccupation. This term applies in FDP when the mother's insistence that her child is ill amounts to an obsession, causing her to ignore all aspects of the child's behavior that do not fit this view.
5. **Corrupting.** Parental behavior that trains the child to be socially deviant, antisocial, or otherwise unfit for normal social experience qualifies for this term. In FDP, corruption will often be found in older children who have been socialized by the mother to cooperate with her in the deception or to initiate factitious illness behavior themselves. Corrupting may be the process by which the mother socially isolates her child and keeps the child as her own possession.

Factitious disorder by proxy is distinguished from other forms of child maltreatment by the fact that third parties are routinely, albeit unknowingly, involved in the abuse. Often most of the physical harm to the child is rendered by doctors through tests, procedures, and medication trials (Meadow 1985, 1989). The term *professional participants* has been used to refer not only to doctors but to legal and child protective personnel who become unwitting participants in the FDP abuse (Zitelli et al. 1987).

The mother's involvement of third parties may be both creative and subtle. She may use the doctor's authority status to justify her insistence that it is bad for the child to play outside in the fresh air with other children. By contriving a medical emergency, she may use doctors to help foil plans for the child to spend time with relatives. Alternatively, she may enlist relatives, friends, and other lay people in socializing the child to play the sick role, especially as the child grows older. Comprehensive assessment in FDP requires understanding the mother's relationship with third parties and the mechanism by which they come to participate in the abuse.

A diagnosis of FDP has significant legal implications because it is a form of child abuse. When diagnosing and evaluating these cases, the physician should follow forensic standards of practice, since expert opinions in the legal context may profoundly affect people's lives (American Psychology-Law Society and Division 41 of the American Psychological Association 1991; American Academy of Psychiatry and the Law 1991). Psychiatric diagnosis is sometimes misused in legal proceedings, where the concern is with whether or not findings of fact conform to specified legal standards, such as those for mental disability or severe physical abuse (American Psychiatric Association 1994; Halleck et al. 1992). When FDP is detected and reported, further psychological evaluation of the mother and/or child is needed to inform the legal decisions that follow.

Comprehensive Individual, Family, and Psychosocial Evaluation Following Detection and Reporting

Factitious disorder by proxy is a diagnosis established by broad examination of comprehensive clinical information, not a characteristic of a mother or child that can be ascertained by individual assessment (Feldman 1994b). Confusion regarding the utility of psychological assessment in FDP arises when an individual assessment model is applied to this complex interpersonal syndrome. The clinical confrontation will often be preceded by some degree of assessment, followed by more in-depth evaluation as needed.

A thorough social, family, and medical history should be obtained, not only from the mother but from collateral sources of information. These include family members, teachers, therapists, doctors, and others. Review of records may include medical and psychiatric records of mother and child as well as police reports, social work reports, the child's school records, depositions, and court transcripts. The history should be studied to decide which episodes of illness are likely to have been fabricated and which were real. In addition, details of the personal, social, and family histories should be confirmed, because the mother may have lied about this information as well.

Letters written by the mother may be reviewed, as well as any audiotapes or videotapes she has made or that have been made of her interacting with the child. Whenever possible, copies should be obtained of the original notes and raw psychological test data of therapists, social workers, and other evaluators involved in the case. Schreier and Libow (1993) describe the findings of a home visit. The mother's living room was decorated with pictures of her child taken years before with tubes coming out of various parts of her body. The mother still carried the child's Broviac catheter, although the child had been removed from her care.

Key behavioral observations of the mother sometimes come from unexpected sources. In the case of Priscilla Phillips, a social worker convicted of murdering the first of her two FDP victims, the observation of a single nurse shattered the "perfect mother" facade. Contrary to the bulk of reports that described Phillips as a wonderful mother, the nurse observed her to be rough and harsh in her handling of the infants (Wright 1984). The child's medical record may contain observations of the mother by doctors and others.

In Case 3, which follows, the mother was repeatedly described in the record as anxious and stressed. These observations contributed to the evaluator's formulation that she belonged to the "perceived illness" subtype of FDP mothers, who express their personal stress and anxiety through overconcern with their children's health. Often they are inexperienced, lonely, or under stress, which makes them more likely to perceive symptoms in their children that others do not observe (Meadow 1985, 1989, 1991). A diagnosis of FDP abuse may be warranted when the mother's behavior is persistent or extreme enough to result in emotional abuse of the child, though conscious maternal deception may not be involved.

Interview of the mother should be viewed as an information-gathering tool, not a lie detector test. Without corroborating information, it is difficult, if not impossible, to ascertain during an interview whether someone is telling the truth (Ford 1996). Careful preparation can enhance the value of information obtained from the interview, for example identifying important questions in advance. The evaluator may wish to ask the mother about events or contradictions in the medical record, information provided by collateral interviews, her relationship with the child, and possible motivations for such behavior.

The power of the psychosocial interview as a data-gathering tool can be further enhanced by use of audio- or videotape. A recorded interview can be reviewed at a later date and shared with colleagues during consultation. If the mother has lied during the interview, recording helps document this behavior; also, an accurate record is kept while eliminating the need to generate concurrent handwritten notes. The interviewer's attention is freed for establishing rapport and for richly exploring relevant lines of inquiry. The evaluator may wish to interview the mother more than once. This effort makes it possible to sample her behavior over time and to pursue questions that may have arisen since the initial interview.

The attempt to establish rapport with the mother maximizes the likelihood that she will cooperate in the assessment. The type and degree of rapport that one develops with her may be relevant to a recommendation for therapy or reunification. Behavioral observations from the interview may suggest themes that can be investigated further. If the mother tends to overwhelm the interviewer with affect, this feature may prompt an exploration of whether she acts this way with the child and with doctors. Such a finding might shed light on the mechanism by which the mother evokes compliance from the child and induces the physician to order more tests. Furthermore, it suggests that physicians and others may need to be briefed in order to manage this maternal style more effectively. In Case 1, which follows, the mother was affectively cold during the interview, unable to establish rapport at all. This observation reinforced the evaluator's opinion that psychotherapy would have limited utility.

The interview provides the most direct opportunity to explore the mother's motivation, although there may be a number of obstacles. She may be unable or unwilling to verbalize her true feelings. Perhaps she is unaware of her motivation, a common feature of factitious disorders (Yorker and Kahan 1991). She may even be quasi-delusional, believing, if only intermittently, that her child is authentically ill. To some extent, the mother's meaningful cooperation in trying to help the interviewer to understand her may be more important than her precise explanation of her behavior.

When exploring the mother's motivation, the physician may follow lines of inquiry suggested by the facts of the case and by familiarity with a variety of motivational profiles. For example, where the facts of a case include prolonged nonattendance at school by a school-age child, the mother's motivational profile may be dominated by her need to keep her child infantalized and dependent. In a different case, which consists primarily of uncomplicated fabrication of seizures, the evaluator might pursue a motivational hypothesis of intense maternal anxiety leading to overconcern with the child's health, as in the perceived illness group of FDP mothers described previously.

Mothers who directly harm their children, poisoning or smothering them, do so for a variety of reasons. Schreier and Libow (1993) view this behavior as a form of maternal risk taking that may be part of a constellation that includes pathological lying and obvious excitement derived from medical crises. When these elements are present, an important motivational hypothesis to pursue is the mother's intense need to engage the child's pediatrician, deriving pleasure from tricking the physician while being viewed by him or her as a "perfect mother." A second motivational picture is suggested in the case reported by Feldman et al. (1989) in which a bulimic mother used ipecac poisoning to induce failure to thrive in her infant. Simultaneously, the mother was becoming emaciated. It appeared that she was treating the child as an extension of herself, imposing her own pathologic need for thinness onto her infant. A third motivational possibility is suggested by Meadow's (1993b) research into a group of FDP salt-poisoning mothers. As noted earlier, retrospective interviews with these women resulted in a gradual admission of feelings of hating their children or wishing them dead.

Being the mother of a sick child can play an important role in the mother's relationship with husband, family, friends, and colleagues. Her ability to gratify her needs by presenting her child in the sick role may help maintain the homeostasis of an unhappy marriage. She may use her expertise in the child's medical problems as a justification to limit the involvement of the husband and others in the child's life. Factitious disorder by proxy may bring the mother closer to her own mother or enable her to compete more successfully with her siblings for their mother's attention. The possible interpersonal benefits of FDP are endless.

A mother may gratify her dependency needs by simultaneously engaging the child's pediatrician and keeping the child enmeshed with her (Folks 1995). In addition, she may gratify intrapsychic needs to see herself as a "better" mother than she has the inclination or skills to be. Meadow (1982) has concluded that it is naive to seek a single cause for FDP. In all probability, the motivation is overdetermined.

The interview provides an excellent opportunity to assess the mother's ability to transcend her self-absorption and talk about her child as a person independent from herself. To this end, the interviewer may wish to determine whether the mother is able to focus her attention on questions about normal developmental milestones and the child's relationships with friends and family. If the child has been socially isolated, it is a good idea to find out whether the mother perceives this isolation as a problem.

Mothers who engage in FDP are often described as selfish and incapable of empathy. This may be less true in cases of FDP in which the emotional abuse is relatively mild and physical abuse is absent. The extent to which there is parental capacity for empathy and loving interpersonal relationships, not just with the child but with others, may provide the basis for recommending therapy for the mother as part of a reunification plan. In assessing capacity for empathy, it would be appropriate to ask the mother what she felt, did, and thought as her child underwent various painful tests and procedures, having her go into some detail. This report can be checked against the observations of collateral sources. Is the mother described by others as holding her child's hand and tearful as he or she screamed, or was she off to the side, chatting with a tech? Descriptions of her actual behavior, as in the Phillips case above, are more useful than nonspecific comments such as, "She was a concerned mother."

Families in which psychological maltreatment occurs often

have few outside supports (Garbarino et al. 1987). This dimension can be assessed in the course of taking the social and family history. Is the mother currently or periodically alienated from her family of origin? Alternatively, is her family part of the problem, reinforcing isolation of the mother-child dyad from the rest of society? Interviewing family members can serve several functions, including assessing the suitability of relatives as potential child guardians. How would the mother's relationships with others be characterized according to such measures as dependence vs. autonomy, mutuality vs. exploitiveness, and stability vs. instability? Where negative interpersonal patterns emerge, the evaluator may wish to explore whether they are ego syntonic.

Often an important part of the assessment will be the mother's persistence in attempting to control interpersonal relationships with physicians, the child, and others. Neale and colleagues (1991) found that case management and child adjustment to placement were adversely affected when mothers persisted in attempting to govern their children even after the FDP was exposed. Many FDP mothers will demonstrate their manipulative, overcontrolling interpersonal style in the interview itself. Other sources of information may be even more revealing of this tendency; for example, the record may show that an FDP mother has used adult factitious disorder as a vehicle to control others.

The extent to which mothers with FDP try to control the pediatrician varies. Mothers who exaggerate or engage in simple fabrications are less controlling than those who sociopathically combine elaborate lies with repeated physical harm and who alter medical records or laboratory findings. There is a significant difference between overanxious mothers who inform the present physician of previous medical contacts and the actively deceptive mothers who hide this information.

Maternal efforts to control physicians may be obscured when a mother accused of FDP is held responsible for physician decisions that were based on factors unrelated to maternal deception. The doctor may know that tests were done at a prior facility but find it easier to repeat the tests than to wade through previous medical records, although the expansion of managed care is discouraging physicians from duplicative testing. In his introduction to Schreier and Libow's 1993 book, Meadow describes the modern doctor as much more likely to order tests or to make referrals to specialists than to spend time listening to the mother and trying to sort out her account. This type of physician orientation needs to be considered or it may lead to overestimation of the mother's active role in influencing physician decisions.

Where the mother's control of the child is concerned, this may be "primary" or "secondary." Control of the child is primary when, for example, a mother with FDP concocts medical justifications for placement of detailed restrictions on her child's eating, sleeping, and eliminating. Here, control appears to be an end in itself. Control of the child may also be primary when the mother uses the child's illness as an excuse to keep the child isolated socially. This type of control obstructs the child's normal development for the purpose of meeting the mother's needs. When present, it helps to define the features of the mother's behavior that are emotionally abusive. On the other hand, control of the child may be secondary, as when the child is used as an object or tool in the mother's plan to manipulate the physician.

Control may be the dominant feature in all of the mother's relationships, whether they be with the child, the physician, the husband, or others. The child is controllable by virtue of his or her dependence and the mother's primary role as the gatekeeper for socialization. A physician or a husband, however, may be actively chosen for qualities that she can manipulate. These characteristics might include the physician's strong desire to be thorough or the husband's passivity and dependence. If she will undertake and participate only in relationships that she can control, then therapy is likely to be dominated by this tendency as well, defeating the purpose of therapy for these women.

Psychological Testing of the Mother

According to Schreier and Libow (1993, p. 164), "Mental health professionals who perform court-ordered assessments of [FDP] parents without the aid of psychological tests—projective tests in particular (tests that assess less conscious psychological material)—are at major risk for being deceived by the parent's often skillfully maintained facade of normalcy." Behind the facade, parents with FDP may have significant psychological problems (Bools et al. 1994), although they may try to conceal this dysfunction when they take psychological tests, as they do elsewhere. Efforts to identify a single test profile that is representative have been unsuccessful. However, characteristics that do seem to emerge with some frequency include superficial social skills, outgoing behavior, poor abstract reasoning ability, and limited stores of information (except for medical knowledge). Psychological test results of mothers with FDP sometimes reveal a rigid, denying defensive style that masks self-centeredness, emotional immaturity, underlying rebelliousness, lack of social conformity, and intense passive resentment (Schreier and Libow 1993).

Psychological testing helps to answer questions about the parent's overall psychological functioning, capacity to parent, and prognosis for responding to different levels of intervention. This information, often important for case planning, is not contained in the diagnosis of FDP alone. Psychological tests provide a standardized means of assessment in contrast to the interview, which varies considerably from one examiner to another. Computer analysis of responses increases the quantity and accuracy of information that can be gained from psychological tests. This type of analysis is available for the Minnesota Multiphasic Personality Inventory (MMPI), Millon Clinical Multiaxial Inventory (MCMI-II), and Rorschach Inkblot Test. Reports generated by computer may suggest diagnostic possibilities that would not have been considered otherwise. Clinical and historical information obtained elsewhere should be used to determine the merit of test-generated statements and hypotheses.

Paper/pencil instruments such as the MMPI and MCMI-II enable the test taker to exert more conscious control over his or her answers, since the examinee is presented with the choice of answering true or false to various statements. Projective measures, however, are more likely to elicit material that is not under conscious control. These measures include the Rorschach, Thematic Apperception Test (TAT), Draw-A-Person (DAP), and Incomplete Sentences. Of this group, only the Rorschach, scored with the Exner system, is sufficiently standardized to meet the threshold of reliability and validity required in legal proceedings.

Once scored, the tests may be laid out and studied for any patterns or inconsistencies across measures. For example, every test might have been taken with extreme defensiveness. This pattern is distinguished from the moderate defensiveness that is common during forensic assessment and might indicate skill at deception, rigid psychological defenses, or an unusually strong refusal to cooperate in the assessment process. Examples of test results and the conclusions drawn from them are presented below.

Case 1

A mother with FDP was highly defensive in taking the MMPI and MCMI-II. Test results showed that she claimed to be unrealistically virtuous, felt inadequate in social situations, and was subject to low moods. A diagnosis of Obsessive Compulsive Personality Disorder with prominent Narcissistic and Aggressive (Sadistic) Personality Traits was suggested. The examiner interpreted these findings to mean that supportive therapy might temporarily relieve the mother's bouts of depression but was unlikely to alter the underlying character problems that put her children at risk for physical and emotional abuse.

Case 2

On the Rorschach, this mother exhibited mild problems with reality testing. Also, she elaborated on her responses by relating them to personal experiences that she described to the examiner. This type of comment indicated that her narcissistic preoccupation leaked into her relationships with others and interfered to some extent with her reality testing. Her highly defensive MMPI suggested that her psychological defenses were both intact and entrenched, probably masking the nature and extent of her pathology. Her drive to be perfect in all things enabled her to ward off narcissistic injury and to feel in control of her world. The FDP behavior forced physicians to recognize what a "perfect" mother she was. It also helped her to control her children, thwarting any efforts at autonomy that might threaten her perfect world.

Case 3

The mother's defenses were found to be inconsistent across tests. They were intact on the MMPI but failed on the Rorschach, where she produced too many responses, a number of them poor in form quality, with a few that even showed cognitive slippage. These findings suggested that she was highly anxious and had the capacity to function well at times, but her defenses were only intermittently effective. When overwhelmed by affect, her perceptions were adversely influenced by her emotional state such that her reality testing was impaired. According to the test results, FDP seemed to be a function of the mother's efforts to manage her anxieties, which included fear of not being a good mother and of losing her child to a possible but unlikely medical condition.

Case 4

This mother's level of psychosocial functioning had degenerated over the years such that she was on disability and had become increasingly socially isolated. She produced a highly defensive MMPI with clinically significant elevations on Psychopathic Deviancy and Mania (4–9 profile). This pattern suggested antisocial tendencies, which were confirmed by other data. The mother was not a candidate for therapy, and emotional abuse was likely to continue if the children were to return to her. Nevertheless, the court offered the mother therapy and allowed the children to return, and the mother reoffended.

Assessing the Mother-Child Interaction

Although mothers with FDP are known for their ability to appear as good mothers, closer examination of the mother-child interaction will often reveal intrinsic disturbances (Roth 1990). Observations from over 200 cases (Neale et al. 1991) identified the following characteristics: the mother-child interaction may appear close, but it is actually overcontrolled by the mother; the mother may be overly dependent on her child; she may treat her children inappropriately for their ages; and/or there may be important discrepancies between the mother's public and private behavior. The presence of these features can be assessed by gathering information from collateral sources and/or observing the mother and child together, even when the child is very young.

One mother, observed with her 9-month-old infant several years prior to the detection of FDP, was described as follows:

> As mother and baby entered the playroom, baby looked at the examiner with curiosity, but the mother missed the cue and did not introduce the baby or promote social involvement. Throughout the observation, mother seemed unable to follow the baby's lead. The mother engaged in much anxious activity with her infant, with many sudden shifts in activity. She initiated a great deal of close physical contact, some of it caregiving in nature, for

> example adjusting the baby's clothing. However, much of it seemed designed to keep the baby close to her and to control the child's interaction with both the mother and the examiner.

It was not until the child was 4 years old that FDP was identified, at which time evaluation of the case revealed the additional finding that the child continued to sleep with her mother.

With children between 3 and 6 years, asking the mother to assist her child in creating a family drawing requires her to enlist the child's cooperation in a task in which the child has no investment. One FDP mother of a 4-year-old boy simply drew the family picture herself. When the examiner encouraged her to work with her son in creating a drawing, she resisted, saying that the child was not a good artist. The mother of a 3-year-old victim of FDP was unable to organize the task at all. She spoke to her daughter using concepts that were much too advanced for her and was unable to see to it that the task was carried out, despite repeated instructions and encouragement from the evaluator. Each mother was unable to cooperate effectively with the examiner, although for different reasons. The first mother insisted on taking over the task, whereas the second mother could not exercise enough adult guidance to accomplish the task.

During the interview of an FDP mother with her two older children present, the interviewer's line of questions that pertained to social isolation were fielded by the children, who described participation in a church youth group and other activities with peers. The evaluator wisely attempted to verify these claims, only to learn that the children had engaged in distortions and fabrications, seemingly to prevent the interviewer from fully grasping the isolation of their family group. Interviewing older children with their mothers can also help determine whether they suffer from shared paranoid disorder, formerly called *folie à deux.*

Another theme for investigation is the degree to which the mother and child have difficulty allowing or tolerating separation, which is a known psychological sequela of FDP abuse. Thus, simply asking to meet with the child alone while the mother remains in the waiting room creates a situation that tests both the child's ability to separate and the mother's response to it. It is not uncommon for a mother with FDP to try to persuade the examiner to allow her to be in the room with the child at all times.

Sometimes the child's medical record will reveal spontaneous, noteworthy observations of the mother-child interaction. In the case of one mother and her son, the doctor recorded that he had admonished the mother after he observed her speaking to the 5-year-old boy in "baby talk." He also noted her insistence on dressing the boy after the medical exam, rather than letting the boy dress himself. In another case, information provided by collateral sources revealed that a 9-year-old girl, the only child of a single mother, had been sleeping with her mother since birth. This practice served to keep the child dependent and to make her available at all hours of the night as her mother's adult confidante. The child experienced her relationship with her mother as ego syntonic, but in different scenarios the child might show more overt signs of stress.

Assessing the Child

Little has been written about psychological assessment of children victimized by FDP. Action plans for protecting such children focus, as they should, on ensuring that the child is in a safe environment. Some information is available, however, about the psychosocial sequelae of FDP abuse. Child victims of FDP abuse are often found to be immature, to have symbiotic relationships with their mothers, and to have separation problems. Infants sometimes develop feeding disorders, apparently in response to unpleasant feeding interactions. Children may display irritability, aggressiveness, and inattention (McGuire and Feldman 1989). A 2½-year-old victim of FDP was reported to exhibit autistic-like behavior when he was first removed from his mother's custody (Porter et al. 1994). His mother had been caught inducing heart failure and was suspected of puncturing his ear drums; in addition, she had created a perforation of the esophagus either by using a foreign object or by inducing severe retching and vomiting. Eighteen months after he was taken into foster care, he experienced a transient psychotic episode. This severely abused child also engaged in what appeared to be reenactment behavior, attempting to suffocate a foster sibling with a pillow, inserting a wire into the ear of a pet dog, and attempting to hang the dog by its leash.

Older children have usually been socialized to "participate" in the deception, so that either the mother or the child may initiate an episode of illness-related trickery with which the other then goes along (Meadow 1984, 1985; Neale et al. 1991). Thus, it is not surprising that older child victims of FDP may develop factitious disorder themselves or other forms of deceptive, manipulative behavior. Sneed and Bell (1976) reported on the case of a 10-year-old boy who inserted small stones into his urethra to simulate the passage of renal stones. In the parlance of child maltreatment, this is an example of a child who has been deeply "corrupted." In the end, child victims of FDP may become psychologically, if not physically, disabled (Meadow 1984, 1985). Generally, the younger the child at the time of intervention, the fewer his or her psychological problems.

Psychological and behavioral sequelae have been found to persist long after the FDP abuse has been identified and the child removed, as the case reported by Porter et al. (1994) demonstrates. About half the children studied by Bools et al. (1993) had conduct and emotional disorders, including problems related to school, attention, and concentration, whether or not they were still living with their mothers at the time of follow-up assessment. (See Chapter 6 for related information.)

Evaluation of the child at the time FDP is detected can help determine the immediate and long-term effects on the child, as well as provide a view of the child's overall social and intellectual development. An example of immediate effects can be seen in a child victim who is generally hyperactive and aggressive but who responds to medical procedures by remaining passive. Hyperactivity may be a form of behavioral arousal caused by the stress of the abuse, whereas passivity during medical procedures may represent a form of accommodation to the abuse. The diagnostic picture may be complicated by the fact that a symptom such as hyperactivity can be due to a genetically influenced biological problem such as attention-deficit/hyperactivity disorder. In general, a causal link between the FDP abuse and the child's psychological symptoms can be more readily established when the mother has been psychologically evaluated and the exact nature and extent of the emotional and/or physical abuse are known.

Depending on the child's age and other factors, techniques for evaluating the child include the following: information from collateral sources, behavioral observation of the child, interview, and psychological testing. Behavioral checklists, a number of which are described by Garbarino and colleagues (1987), allow for systematic collection of data about the child's developmental, behavioral, and social functioning, especially as compared with other children of the same age. Several of these checklists are designed specifically for infants. Behavioral checklists completed by parents and others provide a composite view of the child. The mother's completed checklist can be compared with that of collateral sources. Assessment of the child allows the examiner to learn more about the child's perception of self, his or her mother, and others. To what extent has the child incorporated being sick into his or her self concept? If other aspects of the assessment have identified elements of emotional abuse such as maternal "ignoring" or rejection, the child's perceptions of and response to these maternal behaviors can be explored during an individual interview. For example, has a young boy internalized his mother's treatment of him, feeling bad about himself? Does he comply with the sick role in an effort to make the mother pay more attention to him? If it is known that the child and his mother play a "game of tricking the doctor," interviewing the child alone gives the examiner an opportunity to ask the child what this is all about. In two cases mentioned previously, where the child victims of FDP were still sleeping with their mothers at ages 4 and 9, respectively, the girls might have been asked about their understanding of this unusual sleeping arrangement. Interviewing the child may bring to light relevant behavior of others in the environment, for example a father who is emotionally unavailable by virtue of his drinking or a relative who seems to be colluding with the mother in reinforcing the child's compliance with the sick role.

The child may also be interviewed together with someone besides his or her mother, such as a sibling. For example, in a case where the suspicion of FDP was just beginning to emerge with respect to a 7-year-old boy, he was interviewed with his 4-year-old brother. The interview revealed that the younger child might be feigning seizures: when the interviewer asked the older child about his health, the younger boy leaned over and whispered in the examiner's ear, "Do you want me to show you face wiggling?" He then proceeded to display what appeared to be an imitation of a seizure. The older boy commented wryly, "My brother lies like that all the time." In the interview, the younger child had initiated this sequence to divert the examiner's attention from his older brother. This effort raised questions for further inquiry. Was the younger child simulating illness at home to compete with his older brother for maternal attention? Additionally, was the mother's preoccupation with her children's health being fueled by the younger child's feigning illness, of which the mother was unaware? As part of a comprehensive assessment, the examiner might meet subsequently with the mother, bringing the younger boy's feigned seizure behavior to her attention to test her response.

The use of behavioral observation is illustrated in the case of a 9-year-old girl. Although the child had been subjected to moderate FDP-type emotional abuse for a number of years, it was not until an acute episode of abuse that a mental health professional called child protective services. Of immediate concern was the fact that the mother had contacted scores of people alleging that her child was suicidal. The social worker who took the report decided to observe the child at school, where the girl appeared to be cheerful, though she was on the social fringe of her peer group. Social isolation rather than suicidality seemed to be a problem. Her odd manner of dress and her crudely chopped hairdo also suggested a degree of neglect. When the social worker spoke with the child, her impressions that the child was neither depressed nor suicidal were confirmed.

Psychological testing becomes increasingly feasible with children from age 3 on. There are only a few reports in the literature of psychological test results for child victims of FDP. Testing with children should include measures for both intellectual and emotional functioning. Overall intellectual functioning may be measured using the Wechsler Intelligence Scale for Children (WISC) or the Stanford Binet. Peculiarities of the child's test-taking attitude may be significant, as when a child is unusually afraid to answer for fear of making a mistake. After a teenage girl was removed from her mother because of FDP abuse, her WISC results from age 10 were made available to the evaluator. She had great intellectual potential as measured by six subtests, including those for abstract reasoning. However, relatively speaking, she showed significant impairment on the subtests that measure social perception and general fund of knowledge. These findings were taken as evidence that the years of psychological maltreatment, before the FDP abuse was identified, had adversely affected her intellectual development.

Adolescent victims of FDP can be given the MCMI-II or the MMPI, which are paper-pencil tests with a true-false format. Of the projective tests, the Rorschach, as suggested earlier, has the greatest potential to yield valid, reliable information about the child's overall mental status. The Rorschach protocols of two teenagers, both removed from their mother's custody on an emergency basis, showed marked differences despite the fact that they were siblings. Although both children had been victims of FDP by their mother, the 16-year-old boy had been subjected to additional abuse, in the form of "terrorizing" by an adult relative in the home. Results of his Rorschach showed that he had decompensated under the stress, with loosening of associations and impairment of reality testing. His younger sister, however, had allied herself with the adult terrorizer and acted as her "assistant." Consequently, her defenses, as measured by the Rorschach, were largely intact.

The DAP procedure can provide a measure of the child's developmental mastery of human figure drawings, for which there are norms according to age. The case report of a 4½-year-old victim of FDP compared the girl's drawings of herself before and after intervention (Senner and Ott 1989). Prior to intervention, her drawing of herself was a scribble, chaotic and formless, like that of a 2-year-old. After a brief but intensive nursing intervention in the hospital, she produced a developmentally normal picture that included a head, eyes, and limbs. A 9-year-old girl, asked to draw her family, unconsciously reversed the labels for her mother and herself. Along with other data, this finding was interpreted as demonstrating the lack of psychological differentiation between mother and child (Kahan and Yorker 1991). Depending on the child's age, projective activities such as the DAP, Children's Apperception Test (CAT), Thematic Apperception Test, and Incomplete Sentences can be a useful source of clinical data, although they are not well standardized.

Case Planning

Once FDP is detected, a decision must be made as to whether the child should remain with the mother or be removed. Severe physical abuse or the reasonable risk of it may justify a decision to remove the child. Severity of the emotional abuse, judged in part by the child's behavior, may also warrant such a decision. Where the mother has a history of moving through different communities seeking medical care, this itinerancy may give rise to concerns that she will try to flee the jurisdiction with the child. Additional factors to consider in child placement decisions include whether the mother herself has a documented history of factitious disorder, drug or alcohol dependence, or other mental disorder. A history indicating that other children in the family have suffered abuse, neglect, or death from unknown causes is associated with further abuse and increased risk of morbidity in the index case (Bools et al. 1992). Ostfeld and Feldman note other concerns in Chapter 6.

The advantages and disadvantages of precipitously removing the child from the mother must be considered. Child safety and effective, coordinated case management are among the advantages. Disadvantages include emotional trauma for the child and the lost opportunity to explore the efficacy of less radical interventions first. Once the child has been removed, there tends to be a presumption that such a step was the best course of action, that lesser interventions would not have worked, and therefore that they should not be explored in the future as part of a reunification plan. If the child is allowed to remain with the mother but she persists in fabrications after some degree of confrontation, the child may be removed at that time.

A decision about emergency placement of the child with relatives must likewise balance issues of ensured child protection with those of minimizing trauma for the child by placing him or her with people to whom the child, but also possibly the mother, is attached. An early assessment may need to be made as to whether relatives who might care for the child are sufficiently free of emotional problems themselves. They must be able to accept education about FDP and to adequately protect the child from further physical and/or emotional abuse by the parent with FDP.

Other justifications that have been used for short-term placement of the child away from the mother include helping the child to begin to establish some independence from his or her mother and teaching the child that he or she is not ill. A study by Bools and colleagues (1993) found that children who were temporarily placed in foster care before being returned to their mothers were more likely to have acceptable outcomes at long-term follow-up. It may be that for some mothers, under some circumstances, such a break is therapeutic in ways that are not yet understood.

This section contains other material supplemental to that presented in Chapter 6, including therapy for the mother as a component of the case management plan, for example as a precondition to reunification. Therapy may be contraindicated for a variety of reasons. Even if offered the opportunity, the mother may not be interested in therapy. If she is not, then court-ordering her to participate in therapy is unlikely to be successful and may even delay implementation of more effective interventions, such as permanent placement with another family. There is some controversy among professionals about the need for the mother to admit to the FDP behavior in order to demonstrate a sincere desire for help. Unfortunately, the public censure that comes into play when FDP is detected may intensify the mother's denial. In an effort to ward off being publicly exposed as a liar and abuser, the mother may respond by vigorously maintaining her version of events (Feldman 1994a). If other prognostic indicators are favorable, it may be sufficient that the mother expresses a desire for help even while not admitting to the FDP behavior. Therapy may provide a safer context for the mother to examine her motives and behavior than the often-prescribed confrontation.

In addition to motivation, other positive prognostic indicators for therapy include capacity to establish rapport; logistical capacity to maintain a long-term therapeutic relationship; ability to speak honestly; enough ego strength to accept feedback from the therapist; and capacity to integrate that feedback into insight and behavior change. It may be necessary to have the mother in therapy for several months before all of these dimensions can be adequately assessed. Negative indicators include pathological lying; antisocial or schizoid features; evidence of delusional thinking; fragile defense structure or defenses that are extremely rigid; and a marked tendency to project blame onto others.

There needs to be some agreement between the authorities and the mother about what the therapy should consist of and what its goals should be. If the therapy is too nondirective, the mother will take control of it the way she does in other social relationships, so that it will become a repeat of maladaptive patterns rather than a new learning experience. The therapist must actively structure the therapy and adhere to a well-thought-out treatment plan. The mother must be able to master her control issues enough to comply with the parameters of treatment set by the therapist. These parameters include the mother's signing releases, as is typically specified in the court order, so that the therapist can communicate freely with others involved in the case.

If the child is in placement, further assessment may be needed to determine frequency, duration, and extent of supervision of maternal visits. If the mother has been caught or reasonably suspected of inducing symptoms in her child, visits should be supervised. The extent of the emotional abuse and the mother's ability to control herself may warrant limited but supervised contacts or no contact at all. Where she disrupts the child's placement by creating constant problems, any access permitted will need to be restricted even further. On the other hand, a decision to liberalize the mother's visitation might be based in part on her cooperation with the access program. Her ability to handle appropriately an increase in visitation and removing of supervision restrictions may be an important part of the ongoing assessment as to the potential success of reunification.

Perhaps the primary question in long-term planning is whether the case can be managed adequately if the child remains with, or is returned to, the mother. In an ideal world, "managed adequately" would mean that the child will have an opportunity to grow and develop normally. It also means that the proposed interventions will have a reasonable likelihood of protecting the child from physical, emotional, and medical abuse. For young children who have been subjected to severe abuse, a permanency plan that excludes the mother will usually be most appropriate. Placement of severely abused older children can be more problematic. If the child is deeply attached to his or her mother and has begun in essence to "collude," poor socialization may be so far advanced that placement in a healthier environment does not have the desired positive effect.

In addition to the risk factors contributing to a decision for short-term placement, the following factors point to a poor prognosis for long-term placement with the mother: the mother is unable/unwilling to cooperate with the authorities; the mother continues her fabrications despite some degree of confrontation; and the mother continues her overdependence, overinvolvement, and overcontrol with her child despite intervention attempts. A concise list of conditions that should be met before reunification is carried out appears in the final section of Chapter 6.

Conclusion

By conceptualizing FDP as a complex form of emotional abuse, professionals should find it easier to evaluate, treat, and manage cases in which the child is obviously being harmed, but either there is no physical abuse or the physical abuse cannot be proved.

References

American Academy of Child and Adolescent Psychiatry: Guidelines for the clinical evaluation of child and adolescent sexual abuse. J Am Acad Child Adolesc Psychiatry 27:655–657, 1988

American Academy of Psychiatry and the Law: Ethical Guidelines for the Practice of Forensic Psychiatry. American Academy of Psychiatry and Law Membership Directory, Bloomfield, CT, 1991

American Psychiatric Association: Diagnostic and Statistical Manual of Mental Disorders, 4th Edition. Washington, DC, American Psychiatric Association, 1994, p xxiii

American Psychology-Law Society and Division 41 of the American Psychological Association: Specialty guidelines for forensic psychologists. Law and Human Behavior 15:655–665, 1991

Bools CN, Neale BA, Meadow SR: Co-morbidity associated with fabricated illness (Munchausen syndrome by proxy). Arch Dis Child 67:77–79, 1992

Bools CN, Neale BA, Meadow SR: Follow up of victims of fabricated illness (Munchausen syndrome by proxy). Arch Dis Child 69:625–630, 1993

Bools CN, Neale BA, Meadow SR: Munchausen syndrome by proxy: a study of psychopathology. Child Abuse Negl 18:773–788, 1994

Ceci SJ, Bruck M: Suggestibility of the child witness: a historical review and synthesis. Psychol Bull 113:403–439, 1993

Feldman MD: Denial in Munchausen syndrome by proxy: the consulting psychiatrist's dilemma. Int J Psychiatry Med 24:121–128, 1994a

Feldman MD: The detection of factitious disorder by proxy. Paper presented at the annual meeting of the American Psychiatric Association, Philadelphia, PA, May 1994b

Feldman K, Christopher D, Opheim K: Munchausen syndrome/bulimia by proxy: ipecac as a toxin in child abuse. Child Abuse Negl 13:257–261, 1989

Folks DG: Munchausen's syndrome and other factitious disorders. Neurol Clin 13:267–281, 1995

Ford CV: Lies! Lies!! Lies!!! The Psychology of Deceit. Washington, DC, American Psychiatric Press, 1996, pp 197–220

Garbarino J, Guttmann E, Seeley JW: The Psychologically Battered Child: Strategies for Identification, Assessment and Intervention. San Francisco, CA, Jossey-Bass, 1987

Halleck SL, Hoge SK, Miller RD, et al: The use of psychiatric diagnoses in the legal process: task force report of the American Psychiatric Association. Bull Am Acad Psychiatry Law 20:481–499, 1992

Kahan B, Yorker BC: Munchausen syndrome by proxy: clinical review and legal issues. Behav Sci 9:73–83, 1991

McGuire TL, Feldman KW: Psychologic morbidity of children subjected to Munchausen syndrome by proxy. Pediatrics 83:289–292, 1989

Meadow SR: Munchausen syndrome by proxy. Arch Dis Child 57:92–98, 1982

Meadow R: Munchausen by proxy and brain damage. Dev Med Child Neurol 26:672–674, 1984

Meadow SR: Management of Munchausen syndrome by proxy. Arch Dis Child 60:385–393, 1985

Meadow R: ABC of child abuse: Munchausen syndrome by proxy. BMJ 299: 248–250, 1989

Meadow SR: Commentary: compliance with treatment in asthma and Munchausen syndrome. Arch Dis Child 66:960, 1991

Meadow R: False allegations of abuse and Munchausen syndrome by proxy. Arch Dis Child 68:444–447, 1993a

Meadow SR: Non-accidental salt poisoning. Arch Dis Child 68:448–452, 1993b

Neale B, Bools C, Meadow R: Problems in the assessment and management of Munchausen syndrome by proxy abuse. Children and Society 5:324–333, 1991

Porter GE, Heitsch GM, Miller MD: Munchausen syndrome by proxy: unusual manifestations and disturbing sequelae. Child Abuse Negl 18:789–794, 1994

Rand DC: Munchausen syndrome by proxy as a possible factor when abuse is falsely alleged. Issues in Child Abuse Accusations 1:32–34, 1989

Rand DC: Munchausen syndrome by proxy: integration of classic and contemporary types. Issues in Child Abuse Accusations 2:83–89, 1990

Rand DC: Munchausen syndrome by proxy: a complex type of emotional abuse responsible for some false allegations of child abuse in divorce. Issues in Child Abuse Accusations 5:135–155, 1993

Roth D: How "mild" is mild Munchausen syndrome by proxy? Isr J Psychiatry Relat Sci 27:160–167, 1990

Schreier HA, Libow JA: Hurting for Love: Munchausen by Proxy Syndrome. New York, Guilford, 1993

Senner A, Ott MJ: Munchausen syndrome by proxy. Issues Compr Pediatr Nurs 12:345–357, 1989

Sneed RC, Bell RF: The Dauphin of Munchausen: factitious passage of renal stones in a child. Pediatrics 58:127–130, 1976

Wright NM: A Mother's Trial. New York, Bantam Books, 1984

Yorker BC, Kahan BB: The Munchausen syndrome by proxy variant of child abuse in the family courts. Juvenile and Family Court Journal 42:51–58, 1991

Zitelli BJ, Seltman MF, Shannon RM: Munchausen's syndrome by proxy and its professional participants. Am J Dis Child 141:1099–1102, 1987

CHAPTER 8

Legal Issues in Factitious Disorder by Proxy

Beatrice Crofts Yorker, J.D., R.N., M.S.

The recognition of factitious disorder by proxy (FDP) as a form of child abuse has produced a variety of legal concerns. Most prominent is the need to understand the child abuse reporting laws in each state. No laws have yet created a specific FDP category of abuse. However, protective services personnel and prosecutors have found existing legislative clauses such as "cruelty to children," "child endangerment," "physical harm," "emotional harm," and related statutory language sufficient to fit the unnecessary medical intervention and bodily assault on children who are victims of FDP.

There are several ways to align the spectrum of FDP with statutory definitions of child abuse. If a perpetrator is operating at Libow and Schreier's (1986) milder end of the spectrum by exaggerating or simulating symptoms to cause unnecessary medical diagnostic testing, this behavior can be described as cruelty to children. A health care provider can explain to child protective officials that repeated needle sticks, surgeries, anesthesia, and insertion of tubes into orifices is abuse of the most horrific kind when performed under circumstances in which clinicians have been misled into believing that these interventions are medically justified. In cases of perpetrators who induce actual illness, behaviors such as poisoning, injecting, and smothering clearly constitute assault and are usually defined as physical abuse.

FDP often causes the child to be removed from normal stimulation and age-appropriate activities. This imposition of relative isolation can also meet the statutory definition of deprivation. The psychological sequelae of FDP, such as the child's developing his or her own factitious disorder, constitute emotional abuse, as described more fully in Chapter 7.

All states have child abuse laws with mandatory reporting language. The laws apply to medical and nursing practitioners who would ordinarily be the first to consider FDP. Health care providers need to know that child abuse laws require reporting even suspected abuse. It is the role of protective services agencies, not the clinician, to prove whether abuse did or did not occur. Despite this general rule, health care providers often find themselves inappropriately called upon by skeptical or uninformed protective social workers and judges to provide proof.

Other legal concerns in FDP involve rules of evidence and criminal procedures. These issues will be explored in depth in subsequent sections within this chapter. Legal commentators have cautioned the health care community regarding the fine line between the need to obtain sufficient evidence of abuse and the need to protect the child. Once hospital personnel suspect FDP, the hospital may be liable for civil lawsuits and payment of damages for not protecting the child if subsequent harm occurs (Melfi 1992).

Legal Cases

There are very few references to FDP, or to the previous term, Munchausen syndrome by proxy, in legal case reports. One reason is that juvenile court proceedings are published in a case reporter only if they have been appealed to a state or federal court. Likewise, criminal proceedings are published only on appeal. Nonetheless, the legal cases that have been reported are summarized as follows.

People v. Phillips

The first criminal case in the United States involved the unsuccessful appeal of a California mother convicted of murder. In *People v. Phillips* (1981), the adoptive mother (a child abuse agency volunteer) was found guilty of murdering one child and willfully endangering the life of another. What is useful to note about the Phillips case is the prosecution's ability to obtain a conviction that held up on appeal with only circumstantial evidence and use of expert testimony describing FDP. The mother maintained her innocence during the trial and even in jail. Despite no eyewitness testimony or video surveillance evidence that the mother had actually harmed either of the children, the prosecution of this case provides an exemplar for others who must rely on circumstantial evidence of FDP. One of the most persuasive pieces of evidence that abuse of the second child had occurred was the similarity of the clinical picture to that of another child in the family who had died previously; at the time, the death had not been recognized as being attributable to FDP. The judge found it remarkable that the two adopted children suffered very similar signs and symptoms of diarrhea, dehydration, and extremely high blood levels of sodium. The evidence used to convict the mother included laboratory tests that confirmed hypernatremia, excessive sodium in the formula prepared by Mrs. Phillips for oral feeding, improvement in the children when not in the mother's care, failure of elaborate diagnostic tests to find a physical cause for the condition, and expert testimony by a psychiatrist that Mrs. Phillips's behavior fit the warning signs described in the literature.

The Phillips case serves as a particularly useful legal precedent because it specifically ruled on appeal that the expert witness did not need to have examined Mrs. Phillips, nor did he need to have treated FDP cases, in order to form the opinion that Mrs. Phillips had this particular condition (Searle 1993).

In re Colin R

This Maryland Juvenile Court case involved a 3-year-old boy who had been repeatedly hospitalized for vomiting, dehydration, high urinary output, and low potassium levels. A kidney biopsy showed abnormal calcium deposits, and this finding alerted physicians to the possibility of a drug-induced cause to his problems. Drug testing revealed diuretics in the child's urine. No diuretics had ever been prescribed, as they would have caused the very symptoms of the child's illness. Doctors then filed a petition with the court asking that the boy be placed in protective custody. After a period of no contact with the mother, the child's urine tested negative for diuretics. At that time an investigator from the sheriff's office obtained a warrant to search the mother's home. Police seized hypodermic syringes and two vials of furosemide (a powerful diuretic) from the dresser drawer in the mother's bedroom (*In re Colin R.* 1985).

The court ruled that Colin was "in need of assistance." However, they returned him to the custody of his parents with protective supervision by the Department of Social Services. Six months later, the court reviewed the case and modified the conditions of supervision. Despite the court's acknowledgement that the father had been unable to stop the mother's action, the child was allowed to remain with his natural parents. The decision that the child was in need of assistance and the orders for protective supervision were affirmed on appeal.

Matter of Jessica Z

The opinion of the Family Court of Westchester County in the case of Jessica Z (1987), a 9-month-old with repeated severe diarrhea, was impressive in that the judge cited nine classic articles from the FDP literature and listed seven key warning signs in support of her finding of abuse. The trial of Jessica's mother consumed 14 days, during which 21 witnesses testified; the witnesses included 12 physicians (2 of whom were board-certified psychiatrists), 2 nurses, 1 psychologist, and Jessica's parents. The resulting conflicting expert testimony illustrates the typical scenario in FDP cases. The mother hired the Chief of Pediatric Gastroenterology at a nearby hospital as one of her expert witnesses. He reviewed the records and examined the child. He then testified that there were other possible causes for the persistent diarrhea, such as diverticula and postoperative adhesions. The court, however, found the treating gastroenterologist's opinion that laxatives were the cause of Jessica's symptoms more persuasive.

The mother's expert psychiatrist examined her but did not review the child's medical records. He agreed with an independent court-ordered psychiatrist that there was no evidence of maternal psychosis; however, he disagreed with the other psychiatrist regarding the diagnosis of FDP. Instead, he stated that his psychiatric training enabled him confidently to assess the mother's truthfulness despite the consensus in the literature about the remarkable deceptive abilities of FDP parents.

The court-ordered psychiatrist had both reviewed the medical records and interviewed the mother and father. He found a "high probability" that the mother caused Jessica to ingest laxatives, thereby inducing her illnesses. He also noted her extraordinarily calm self-assurance and lack of concern over the interview process. The court then cited Waller's (1983) discussion of psychiatric evaluations of mothers with FDP as consistent with the expert reports in this case.

The court further ruled that the following circumstantial evidence was indicative of abuse: laboratory stool tests were positive for the laxative phenolphthalein, a component of Ex-Lax; the day after the staff confronted the mother with the suspicion of FDP, she had apparently surreptitiously placed a bar of Ex-Lax in another child's bottle of formula, then exclaimed to the staff, "This should prove that Mom didn't do it"; and Jessica had been free of symptoms once the mother was removed from her care. The court went on to apply the doctrine of *res ipsa loquitur* (the thing speaks for itself). This doctrine is very useful in FDP cases, as circumstantial evidence is often the only evidence available. It is an appropriate legal principle that applies to the common finding in FDP cases that the child thrives once separated from the perpetrator. The doctrine of *res ipsa loquitor* is derived from tort, or civil, law, and the following elements must be present: 1) the event must be the kind that does not ordinarily occur without someone's negligence or wrongdoing; 2) it must be caused by an agency or instrumentality within the exclusive control of the defendant; and 3) it must not have been due to any voluntary action on the part of the injured party (Prosser et al. 1988). *Res ipsa loquitor* is exemplified by the miraculous recovery of a very ill child once removed from the exclusive control of the alleged perpetrator.

Place v. Place

The Place case (1987) was decided by a New Hampshire Family Court in the same year as the Jessica Z case. This case was distinguished from the others in that it involved a custody dispute between the divorced parents rather than a determination of child abuse by the state.

The appellate court upheld Mr. Place's petition for physical custody of his two daughters, aged 13 and 7. Though both girls preferred to live with their mother, the court found that the mother was "unable to cope with the fact that her [13-year-old] daughter has no objectively determinable symptoms of serious illness" and that the daughter was likely to be subjected to repeated and unnecessary invasive medical investigations if left with the mother. The appellate court agreed with the trial court that the mother was psychologically unfit and a threat to her children. (Table 8–1 summarizes court cases involving allegations of FDP between 1990 and 1994.)

Themes

One positive theme that emerges when one reviews the legal cases is the recognition by the courts that FDP is a form of child abuse. Even on appeal, findings of deprivation are being upheld in the majority of decisions. On the other hand, the most disconcerting finding is that in only 2 of 11 cases were parental rights terminated. In three other cases, however, criminal prosecution of two mothers and one grandmother presumably prevented continued contact with child victims. In three juvenile court cases, reunification was allowed with a period of supervision, whereas in four cases, the outcome was unknown. Perhaps the judicial rationale for supervised reunification was most aptly stated by the judge in the Jessica Z case:

> The risks entailed in leaving the child at home include: 1) illness produced by the perpetrator; 2) illness simulated by the perpetrator; and 3) real illness not treated, due to the family's feeling of being threatened as a result of legal proceedings. Removal of the child to the unknown circumstances of foster care poses other risks. Such an order would result in the child's separation not only from respondent/mother, but from her father, her sibling, and her grandparents. This further disruption of Jessica, who, at 18 months of age has been subjected to such great physical and emotional suffering, would cause her further trauma, and possibly permanent damage. The most prudent course appears to this court to be one which permits Jessica to remain at home, while providing maximum safeguards, such as have been advocated by the professionals who have had experience with FDP

Table 8–1. Factitious disorder by proxy cases in the courts

Case name	Court	Case description	Outcome
Geringer v. Iowa Department of Human Services, 521 N.W.2d 730 (Ia. 1994)	Iowa Supreme Court upheld finding of abuse by Juvenile Court	Mother appealed a judgment upholding an adverse report by the Iowa DHS. A child abuse report had been filed against the mother for "staging baseless vomiting and bleeding incidents" in her daughter. Judgment of the district court affirmed.	Child returned home to mother
In re: White, 1994 WL 6681 (Ohio App. 5 Dist.)	Ohio Court of Appeals	Temporary custody action where the child was taken into custody based on the pediatrician's diagnosis that the mother suffered from FDP. The child had remained in temporary custody for over 1 year. The court determined that the lower court's jurisdiction had expired because the statutory purpose was to prevent "indefinite . . . family disruptions of more than one year. . . ." Judgment reversed.	Outcome unknown
Matter of Jordan, 616 N.E.2d 388 (Ind.2d 1993)	Indiana Court of Appeals, 2nd District	Mother appealed judgment in favor of Marion County DPW. Son was taken into protective custody after DPW received a report alleging mother had FDP. Because of a holiday and court delays, the post-detention hearing was not held for nearly 156 hours. The court determined that this was proper based on the child's best interest. Judgment affirmed.	Outcome unknown

(continued)

Table 8–1. Factitious disorder by proxy cases in the courts *(continued)*

Case name	Court	Case description	Outcome
In Interest of B.B., 500 N.W.2d 9 (Ia. 1993)	Iowa Supreme Court affirmed Juvenile Court decision to place child in foster care	Parents appealed lower court ruling finding their 16-year-old mentally retarded son in need of assistance (foster care and visitation restrictions). District court affirmed the decision based on parents' failure to send son to school and mother's "obsession with child's health."	Child to remain in foster care until 18 years old
State v. De Jesus, 1993 WL 171866 (Conn. Super.)	Connecticut Superior Court upheld trial outcome in Criminal Court	Grandmother pled nolo contendere and was convicted of risk of injury to a minor. The grandmother had brought her grandson to the hospital with "seizures." While he was hospitalized, a nurse witnessed the grandmother fracture the child's leg. Subsequent radiological examinations revealed that the baby had suffered other broken bones. The grandmother argued for a reduction of her sentence, but the court upheld the sentence as reasonable in light of the evidence and the need to protect innocent parties.	Outcome for child unknown; grandmother in jail

In the Interest of M.A.V., 206 Ga. App. 299, 425 S.E.2d 377 (1992)	Georgia Court of Appeals reversed Juvenile Court	Earlier proceedings proving mother's FDP with younger child led to termination of parental rights of older child. (M.A.V. might become the next victim of the mother's FDP.) The court held that the evidence presented did not support termination.	Reversed
Matter of Bowers, 1992 WL 2870 (Ohio App. 4 Dist.)	Ohio Court of Appeals reversed in part Juvenile Court's finding of abuse	ACCS appealed a judgment of failure to prove that the child was neglected or dependent and an order to return the child to the mother's custody. ACCS argued that the child was at risk due to the mother's alleged FDP. The Court of Appeals found sufficient evidence to support the lower court's ruling that ACCS had failed to meet its burden of proof because of conflicting expert testimony about FDP. Reversed in part and remanded for further proceedings.	Outcome unknown
State v. Lumbrera, 252 Kan. 54, 8545 P.2d 609 (1992)	Kansas Supreme Court overturned judgment in Criminal Court trial	Mother appealed jury trial conviction of first-degree murder of her son (death from asphyxia by smothering). Mother's five other children had died young and unattended. One of the state's theories relative to the motive for the homicide was that the mother suffered from FDP. However, the conviction was reversed and the case remanded for a new trial due to cumulative trial errors.	Mother's conviction for murder reversed

(continued)

Table 8–1. Factitious disorder by proxy cases in the courts *(continued)*

Case name	Court	Case description	Outcome
Matter of Tucker, 578 N.E.2d 774 (Ind.4d 1991)	Indiana Court of Appeals upheld Juvenile Court's termination of parental rights	Mother appealed termination of parental rights. The Court of Appeals held that the termination was supported by the evidence and was based in part on mother's mental illness. Testimony at trial indicated that the mother "could have" FDP. Further, the son's emotional state improved and he stopped self-abusive behavior when in foster care.	Parental rights terminated
Commonwealth v. Robinson, 565 N.E.2d 1229 (Mass. App. Ct. 1991)	Massachusetts Appeals Court upheld criminal conviction of involuntary manslaughter	Mother appealed conviction for involuntary manslaughter of her 11-month-old hospitalized child, which resulted from poisoning caused by massive salt intoxication. The prosecutor was barred from introducing any evidence concerning FDP. However, the Appeals Court held that the evidence presented, although circumstantial, supported the conviction.	Mother convicted

In re: S.R., 599 A.2d 364 (Vt. 1991)	Vermont Supreme Court upheld Juvenile Court's termination of both parents' rights	Parents appealed termination of parental rights. Previous smothering by mother led to diagnosis of FDP. The father's drinking problems and both parents' continued denial were considered. The Supreme Court affirmed based on the risk of injury and developmental harm to the child.	Child in pre-adoptive foster home. Free to be adopted

Note. DHS = Department of Human Services; FDP = factitious disorder by proxy; DPW = Department of Public Welfare; ACCS = Athens County Children's Services

> cases, subject to review in six months. Recommendations of others include a plan whereby communication between respondent's psychiatrist and the child's primary physician is assured. This contact is obviously necessary since the child's illness is the only reliable symptom of the mother's disorder.

Another explanation for this trend toward reunification may be found in the recommendations of experts. For example, in Jessica Z's case, her doctor testified that in his past experience with FDP, "confrontation of the mother resulted in her cessation of the abusive conduct." The psychologist agreed. In contrast, a compelling argument for swift termination of parental rights in extreme cases of FDP was made by Kinscherff and Famularo (1991). This paper was published after the Jessica Z testimony that intervention tended to deter further abuse. The authors note that in a number of cases cited by McGuire and Feldman (1989), some accused parents continued to abuse the child even while being supervised (Kinscherff and Famularo 1991; Juvenile Court of Whitfield Co. 1994).

There is a strong legal presumption in favor of parental rights, and termination of these rights requires not only persistent life-threatening or injurious conduct but clear and convincing proof of the parent's inability to be rehabilitated. In the cases of successful termination of parental rights, it has been the parents' persistent failure to abide by the criteria set out by protective services officials that caused this outcome.

Juvenile courts decide matters of dependency. Typically, the state department of child protective services initiates a hearing granting a custody review. The standard of proof in juvenile proceedings is a preponderance of the evidence. Juvenile courts determine plans for protection of the child and examine custody determinations according to the best interests of the child.

Criminal courts prosecute the perpetrators of child abuse and levy statutory sentences for offenders. The standard of proof in a criminal case is beyond a reasonable doubt. Thus, many cases found to be child abuse in juvenile proceedings never result in criminal prosecution because of the great difference in standards of proof.

Family courts deal with issues regarding divorce and custody, as in *Place v. Place* (1987). In some cases, there may be several courts involved: the juvenile court, to rule on the disposition of the child as abused or in need of assistance; the criminal court, to act on any pending criminal charges; and the family court, to hear custody disputes.

Criminal Procedure

Child abuse is just one of the ways in which hospitals are increasingly involved in forensics. Thus, health professionals need to understand rules of criminal procedure and evidence. When a crime is suspected, police or investigative officials will want to gather evidence that is sufficiently strong to meet the high burden of proof beyond a reasonable doubt.

There are several safeguards enumerated in the Constitution and the Bill of Rights for persons suspected of committing a crime. The Fourth Amendment details "the right of the people to be secure in their houses, papers, and effects, against unreasonable searches and seizures." In order to obtain a warrant to search for evidence of a crime, authorities must meet a standard that is much less stringent than that needed to obtain a conviction; officials need to show only probable cause that a crime has been committed. Generally, permission from a magistrate in the form of a warrant should be obtained prior to a search or seizure. The petition for the warrant should specify what area will be searched and what evidence is expected to be found. Three general exceptions to the need for a warrant are searches made during an arrest, searches conducted after the person consents to it, or searches in emergency circumstances. Emergency or exigent circumstances include situations in which a suspect is about to destroy evidence (e.g., removing dried blood from fingernails [*Cupp v. Murphy* 1973]), situations that may endanger others (*People v. Sirhan* 1972), or cases involving "hot pursuit of a suspect" (*Warden Maryland Penitentiary v. Hayden* 1967).

Another exception includes searches that involve no reasonable expectation of privacy, such as searches of garbage (*California v. Greenwood* 1988), things in plain view (*Harris v. U.S.* 1968), or open fields (*Oliver v. U.S.* 1984). Although there have been no published cases in which an FDP perpetrator has claimed that covert video surveillance of his or her actions was unconstitutional and, therefore, inadmissible, *State v. Abislaiman* (1983) can be used to infer judicial support for covert video surveillance. In that case, a police officer set up video surveillance on telephone poles in a hospital parking lot, allowing police observation from an unseen location. At 2:30 A.M., the officer observed a couple drive in and park. He activated the zoom lens on the camera, observing the suspect in the car take a gun from his belt. The police officer then walked over to the car, ordered the couple out, searched the car, and found the gun, marijuana, and methaqualone. The court of appeals ruled that the video surveillance, even the zoom lens, did not violate any reasonable expectation of privacy. The evidence was admissible and the conviction upheld.

Electronic surveillance such as wire tapping (*Katz v. U.S.* 1967) is considered a "search" according to the Fourth Amendment. However, there is sufficient related case law that would imply that a hospital room is not a place that offers a constitutionally protected reasonable expectation of privacy (Kahan and Yorker 1991). Thus, covert video surveillance would presumably be considered admissible evidence (Yorker 1995).

As noted, a warrant is not needed when there is consent for the search. Some hospitals have added a sentence to the consent for treatment form that parents sign upon their child's admission to a hospital that reads, "I consent to the taking and publishing of still or motion pictures of the patient's diagnosis and treatment. In addition, closed circuit television monitoring of patient care may also be used for educational or clinical purposes unless I request otherwise."

Other rulings useful to FDP cases are those that have held that justifiable intrusions into the body do not per se violate the Fourth Amendment. These rulings may be relevant to professionals attempting to confirm suspicions of FDP. In a representative case, a patient suspected of driving under the influence of alcohol protested against having blood drawn for an alcohol level. The court stated that the phlebotomy was not a violation of the patient's Fourth or Fifth Amendment rights (*Schmerber v. California* 1966). Likewise, use of X ray or a stomach pump to obtain evidence of concealed drugs has been upheld (*U.S. v. Montoya de Hernandez* 1985). These rulings lend support to a hospital staff's wishing to obtain medical evidence over parental objections in FDP cases.

Other relevant constitutional provisions include the Fifth Amendment privilege against forced self-incrimination, the Sixth Amendment right to legal assistance, and the Fourteenth Amendment due process clause that has been interpreted to require fundamental fairness in state criminal proceedings (*Duncan v. Louisiana* 1968).

A general rule of criminal procedure is that evidence that is obtained in violation of a person's Fourth, Fifth, or Sixth Amendment rights will be excluded from any subsequent trial (*Mapp v. Ohio* 1961). There is, however, an exception to this exclusionary rule that could apply in a FDP case. The U.S. Supreme Court has held that evidence obtained in violation of a person's constitutional rights by a private party (i.e., one not acting under the direction or employment of a law enforcement agency) is admissible (*Burdeau v. McDowell* 1921). Physicians, nurses, or hospital administrators would most likely qualify as private parties for purposes of the exclusionary rule. Protective services workers may or may not qualify depending on local law.

As indicated, the private party exception is derived from a 1921 case, and, although *Burdeau* has not been directly overruled, state courts have sometimes suppressed evidence obtained through illegal searches by private persons. For example, as discussed by Kahan and Yorker (1991), the Montana Supreme Court held that warrantless searches that invade personal privacy, whether conducted by private persons or government officials, are per se unreasonable (*State v. Hyem* 1981).

Rules of Evidence

Evidence is either direct or circumstantial. Some general rules of evidence are useful to know in the prosecution of FDP. The hearsay rule excludes any statement made by someone other than the witness testifying. A witness cannot testify regarding what someone else said. This limitation stems from the presumption that it is far more reliable to get the person who made a statement to speak for himself or herself. Furthermore, statements made outside the courtroom cannot be held to be as reliable as those made in court, under oath, and with the opportunity for cross-examination.

One of the useful exceptions to the hearsay rule includes statements made to a physician or health professional for the purpose of obtaining "medical diagnosis or treatment" (FRE 803[4]). These statements are generally believed to be reliable; thus, there is no need for exclusion. This particular exception has been most helpful in sexual abuse cases, allowing a treating physician to testify as to what the patient disclosed about the circumstances of a rape.

An additional exception to the hearsay rule that allows health professionals to testify to what the suspect said is any such statement that helps to describe the suspect's "state of mind" (FRE 803[3]). Thus, in the Jessica Z case (1987), the nurse was allowed to testify verbatim to what she heard the mother say about the Ex-Lax in the bottle of formula. This material was used to illustrate the mother's state of mind rather than being held out as an objectively accurate statement; thus, it fit the exception.

Another general exclusion applies to evidence of prior crimes. In general, a suspect is to be tried according to only the evidence of the present crime. This rule is to overcome the tendency to convict a defendant with prior charges based on the assumption that he or she is a "bad person." A very helpful exception to this rule also applies in FDP cases, however. Evidence of a prior crime is admissible if it shows a common plan or scheme or a modus operandi (*Jones v. State* 1965). Information regarding prior sibling deaths (DiMaio and Bernstein 1974; Schreier and Libow 1993) or of prior suspicious deaths in the presence of a particular babysitter (Richardson 1987) have been specifically allowed in prosecutions of FDP. The case of *United States v. Woods* (1973), referenced by DiMaio and Bernstein (1974), involved the prosecution of a woman for the assault and first degree murder of her 8-month-old foster son. The court of appeals ruled that evidence could be admitted showing that 9 other children who had been in the custody of Mrs. Woods had suffered a total of at least 20 episodes of cyanosis. Seven of these children died, and five had experienced multiple episodes of cyanosis. Three of the children were her own natural children, two were children she adopted, one was a niece, one was a nephew, and two were children of friends for whom she was babysitting. In justifying the exception to the general rule of excluding evidence of prior criminal acts, the court of appeals stated, "We think also that when the crime is one of infanticide or child abuse, evidence of repeated incidence is especially relevant because it may be the only evidence to prove the crime" (p. 133).

Direct Evidence

Direct evidence is by far the most persuasive way to meet the proof beyond a reasonable doubt standard. The legal definition of direct evidence is "evidence that resolves a matter in issue" (Cleary and Graham 1984).

Eyewitness observations are examples of direct evidence often used in the prosecution of FDP cases. In several recent cases, nurses have testified that they observed a mother covering the infant's mouth and nose immediately preceding an apnea episode. Another example is a nurse who observed a mother hide wet diapers after reporting that the child was not voiding. Producing the wet diapers would be an example of "real" evidence. Producing a medical record with the weight of the diaper recorded would be "documentary" evidence. Each can be used to support testimonial evidence.

Videotaped recordings provide another example of direct evidence; however, several procedural safeguards apply. First, a foundation must be laid to show how the video recording was made and to ensure there was no editing or tampering. The judge may also exclude parts of the recording that would not be essential to a finding of guilt so as to avoid unnecessary invasion of privacy. As discussed above, there are numerous legal issues associated with closed circuit surreptitious video surveillance as a means of obtaining evidence of FDP. There are also practical issues, outlined in Table 8–2.

Confessions can serve as direct evidence. However, as described in other situations above, there are numerous safeguards that can render confessions inadmissible. If a suspected perpetrator makes statements to a health care provider that tend to incriminate him or her, they would most likely be allowed into evidence. Once the police or other investigative officials are involved and the suspected perpetrator is taken into custody, however, he or she must be notified of the Sixth Amendment right to counsel, the fact that statements made can be held against him or her, and the Fifth Amendment right to remain silent (*Miranda v. Arizona* 1966).

An interesting recent case (*United States v. Welch* 1994) involves a mother's appeal of an FDP conviction. She maintained that her constitutional rights under *Miranda* were violated when a videotaped confession that she had smothered three of her children, killing two, was entered into evidence. As background, a plain clothes detective had invited the mother to the hospital to discuss a false police report she had made shortly after she had been reported to authorities for smothering her third child. The interview room was equipped with a hidden camera and microphones. The mother was told that her presence was voluntary, that she could refuse to answer any questions, and that she could leave any time. She was not read her rights under *Miranda* (which further demands that suspects be informed that what they say may be held against them and that they have the right to legal counsel) until after her confession. The Sixth Circuit Court of Appeals ruled that the mother was not coerced or deprived of her

Table 8–2. Considerations in covert video surveillance

Advantages	Disadvantages
• Provides excellent direct evidence of parental action that harms the child	• Most effective with active inducers who continue to induce the child's illnesses in the hospital
• Can be used during confrontation to encourage a confession	• Can be evaded if mother is suspicious
• Can be shown in court	• Expensive, and less effective with those who falsely report symptoms
• Can be dramatic proof, without using opinion or circumstantial evidence	• Can be difficult to interpret
• May have therapeutic value in treatment of the mother	• Can be thought of as endangering the child if the mother is allowed access to the child to provide video evidence
• Is very useful for medical diagnostic purposes	• Can include damaging information that has no bearing on the possibility of child abuse

liberty, and that a 2-hour interview with hidden surveillance did not constitute an illegally obtained confession. Despite the fact that the police officer "acted like a therapist" and misrepresented information that a new DNA test showed her other children could not have died of sudden infant death syndrome, the judge said it was a validly obtained confession.

Circumstantial Evidence

Often in cases of FDP, there is no direct evidence, yet there is sufficient probable cause to intervene to protect the child. As noted, many of the legal cases reviewed relied on circumstantial evidence for convictions of murder or determinations of abuse.

Perhaps the most powerful circumstantial evidence used in FDP cases is the presence of clinical indicators of illness when the child is in the care of the suspected perpetrator, but remarkable improvement in the child's physical state during and after a period of separation. Demonstrative evidence can be very helpful to the court. These aides might include graphs or tables illustrating severity of symptoms in the presence of the caretaker and establishing a baseline during and after separation. The author recently provided graphs of a victim's weight, medication use, symptoms of illness, school absences, and academic performance. All the indcators dramatically improved after the mother was arrested for forging prescriptions, and the child was placed in foster care (Juvenile Court of Whitfield Co. File No. S:155-93-00543, 1994). Other examples of demonstrative circumstantial evidence include photographs (e.g., of pressure points on the child's neck or pinch marks on the nose).

Any physical or real evidence that is introduced (e.g., syringes, intravenous tubing, or bottles of toxins found in the trash) must be offered with reassurances that the appropriate chain of evidence was followed. This measure will help undermine challenges that evidence has been tampered with or substituted. Generally, toxicologic blood or serologic lab reports are considered admissible evidence. For example, if the blood type of the mother corresponds to blood found in a child's urine or stool specimen and is not the blood type of the child, this finding provides good circumstantial evidence for FDP. Also, as in Phillips, Jessica Z, and

Colin R, serologic studies that reveal presence of a drug that has not been ordered for the child can help persuade the court that poisoning has occurred.

Conclusion

Courts must balance the rights of a defendant with the health and welfare of a potential victim when evaluating the actions of care providers and investigators in child abuse cases. The courts have tended to consider FDP as grounds for a finding of abuse or dependency. However, they have also tended to reunify and supervise rather than terminate parental rights. The potential for backlash against the diagnosis is present in FDP prosecutions, just as in sexual abuse. In England, for example, a group of 12 mothers accused of having FDP, some of whom have been able successfully to appeal the diagnosis, formed a group called Parents Against Injustice. They argue that FDP is simply a "dust bin diagnosis" used by lazy or incompetent physicians who cannot accurately find the cause of their children's problems (Morgan 1993). A recent British law journal contained an article outlining several criticisms of video surveillance, including allegations that it invades privacy rights, does not work cooperatively with families, and may even endanger children while it tries to "catch" offenders (Thomas 1994). Despite these critiques, when considerations of child safety are primary and due process is considered, the legal avenues for acknowledging FDP as a form of abuse in the courts are very promising.

References

Burdeau v McDowell, 256 U.S. 465, 65 LEd 1048, 41 SCt 474 (1921)

California v Greenwood, 486 U.S. 35, 100 LEd2d 30, 108 SCt 1625 (1988)

Cleary EW, Graham MH: Cleary and Graham's Handbook of Illinois Evidence, 4th Edition. Boston, Little, Brown, 1984

Cupp v Murphy, 412 U.S. 291, 36 LEd2d 900, 93 SCt 2000 (1973)

DiMaio VJM, Bernstein CG: A case of infanticide. J Forensic Sci 19:745–754, 1974

Duncan v Louisiana, 391 U.S. 145, 20 LEd2d 499, 88 SCt 1444, (1968)

FedREvid 803(3),(4)(1975)

Harris v U.S., 390 U.S. 234, 19 LEd2d 1067, 88 SCt 992, (1968)

In re Colin R, 493 A2d 1083, (Md App 1985)
Jones v State, 376 SW 2d 842, (Tex 1964)
Juvenile Court of Whitfield Co File No S:155–93–00543 (Ga 1994) (unreported)
Kahan BB, Yorker BC: Munchausen syndrome by proxy: clinical review and legal issues. Behav Sci Law 9:73–83, 1991
Katz v U.S., 389 U.S. 347, 352–35 (1967)
Kinscherff R, Famularo R: Extreme Munchausen syndrome by proxy: the case for termination of parental rights. Juvenile and Family Court Journal 42:41–53, 1991
Libow JA, Schreier HA: Three forms of factitious illness in children: when is it Munchausen syndrome by proxy? Am J Orthopsychiatry 56:602–611, 1986
Mapp v Ohio, 367 U.S. 643, 6 LEd2d 1081, 81 SCt 1684, (1961)
Matter of Jessica Z, 515 NYS 2d 370, 135 Misc 2d 520, (Fam Ct 1987)
McGuire TL, Feldman KW: Psychological morbidity of children subjected to Munchausen syndrome by proxy. Pediatrics 83:289–292, 1989
Melfi MH: Munchausen syndrome by proxy: "please protect me from my parents." Paper presented at the 14th annual conference of the American Society for Healthcare Risk Management, Las Vegas, NV, November 1992
Miranda v Arizona, 384 U.S. 436, 16 LEd2d 694, 86 SCt 1602, (1966)
Morgan B: Letters to the editor. The Independent, May 24, 1993, p 25
Oliver v U.S., 466 U.S. 170, 104 SCt 1735 (1984)
People v Phillips, 122 Cal App3d 69 (1981)
People v Sirhan, 497 P2d 1121 (Ca 1972)
Place v Place, 525 A2d 704 (NH 1987)
Prosser WL, Wade JW, Schwartz VE: Cases and Materials on Torts, 8th Edition. Mineola, NY, The Foundation Press, 1988, pp 241–264
Richardson GF: Munchausen syndrome by proxy. Am Fam Physician 36:119–123, 1987
Schmerber v California, 384 U.S. 757, 86 SCt 1826, 16 LEd2d 908 (1966)
Schreier HA, Libow JA: Hurting for Love: Munchausen by Proxy Syndrome. New York, Guilford, 1993
Searle M. Munchausen syndrome by proxy: a guide for California attorneys. Western State University Law Review 20:393, 1993
State v Abislaiman, 437 So2d 181 (Fla 3d DCA 1983)
State v Hyem, 630 P2d 202 (Mont 1981)
Thomas T: Covert video surveillance. New Law Journal 144:966–967, 1994
U.S. v Montoya de Hernandez, 473 U.S. 531, 105 SCt 3304, 87 LEd2d 381 (1985)
U.S. v Welch, 36 F3d 1098 (SD Ohio 1994)
U.S. v Woods, 484 F2d 127 (4th Cir 1973)

Waller DA: Obstacles to the treatment of Munchausen by proxy syndrome. J Am Acad Child Psychiatry 22:80–85, 1983

Warden Maryland Penitentiary v Hayden, 387 U.S. 294, 18 LEd2d 782, 87 SCt 1642, (1967)

Yorker B: Covert video surveillance of Munchausen syndrome by proxy: the exigent circumstances exception. Health Matrix: Journal of Law—Medicine 5:325–346, 1995

CHAPTER 9

Hospital Epidemics of Factitious Disorder by Proxy

Beatrice Crofts Yorker, J.D., R.N., M.S.

In 1977, when Meadow published his seminal work on factitious disorder by proxy (FDP), an epidemic of suspicious breathing failures in a Michigan hospital was being attributed to two nurses (*U.S. v. Narciso and Perez* 1977). Three years earlier, a nurse in Scotland had been convicted of injecting patients needlessly with insulin (*H.M. Advocate v. McTavish* 1974). Since that time, such epidemics of illnesses induced by nurses have continued to be identified approximately once every 1½ years (Table 9–1).

In 1988, the first systematic investigation of nurses charged with serial murder was published (Yorker 1988), and the link to factitious disorders began to emerge in the author's mind. Since then, the use of FDP as a paradigm for understanding serial murder by health care professionals has been gaining acceptance (Davies 1993; Levin and Sheridan 1995; Repper 1995; Schreier and Libow 1993).

Registered nurses comprise the largest group of professional caregivers associated with serial killings and assaults in hospitals; there are at least 13 documented cases (Yorker 1994). These epidemics are not limited to registered nurses, however. Forrest (unpublished observations 1992) analyzed caregiver-associated serial killings (CASK) and found that medical doctors, pharmacists, osteopaths, and others have been identified as murderers.

Table 9–1. Nurses charged with serial murder in hospitals

Year of case	Location	CDC study?	Suspicious deaths *N*	Counts of *murder* *N*	Counts of *assault* *N*	Conviction?	Unit	Shift	Nurse's age and sex	Confession?	Assault	Psychiatric history?
1974	Scotland	No	23	1	4	Yes, appealed murder conviction and won	Geriatric	?	34, F	No	Insulin injection	Yes
1975	Michigan (2 nurses)	Yes[1]	10	1	3	Yes, appealed and conviction set aside	ICU and floor	3–11	29, F and 30, F	No	Pancuronium bromide injection	No
1981	Canada	Yes[2]	18	4	6	No	Ped. ICU and floor	11–7	?, F	Yes	Digoxin injection	No
1981	California	No	27	12	12	Yes, lost appeal	ICU, CCU	11–7	46, M	No	Lidocaine injection	Yes, FD
1982	Texas	Yes[3]	20	1	0	Yes, lost appeal	Ped. ICU, outpatient ped.	3–11 ICU, day in office	31, F	No	Succinyl-choline injection	Possible MS
1984	Florida	Yes[4]	12	4	0	Yes	Nursing home	11–7	29, F	Yes	Insulin injection	Yes, MS

985 1	Georgia	Yes[6]	10	6	20	Yes, lost appeal	ICU	3–11	23, F	Yes	KCl and clonidine injections	Yes, DD
1985	Maryland	Yes[5]	10	3	7	No	ICU	3–11	31, F	Yes, inadmissable	KCl injection	?
1986	W. Germany	No	17	9	?	Yes	ICU	3-11	31, F	Yes	Chloride of Kalium	?
1987	New York	No	7	1	3	Yes	ICU, cardiology	11–7	27, M	Yes	Pancuronium and succinylcholine injections	?
1992	Florida	No	30	?	?	Yes	ICU, other floors	prn	36, M	No	Lidocaine and epinephrine injections	?
1992	Alabama	No	18	1	?	Yes, appealing	Nursing homes	prn	?, M	Yes	Lethal doses of thioridazine in feeding tubes	?
1993	England	No	4	4	8	Yes	Pediatrics	Varied	23, F	Only after conviction	Insulin, suffocation, and air embolus	Yes, MS

Note. MS = Munchausen syndrome; DD = dissociative disorder; FD = factitious disorder. [1]Stross et al. 1976; [2]Buehler et al. 1985; [3]Istre et al. 1985; [4]Sacks et al. 1988a; [5]Sacks et al. 1988b; [6]Franks et al. 1987. *Source.* Reprinted and adapted with permission from Yorker BC: "An Analysis of Murder Charges Against Nurses." *Journal of Nursing Law* 1:35–46, 1994.

Linedecker and Burt (1990) describe 10 nursing aides convicted of serial murder, and the literature on fatal FDP includes other paid caregivers, such as babysitters, as perpetrators.

In addition, providers of direct care are not the only occupational groups to be linked to factitious disorders. Firefighters have started fires in order to be heroes (Levin and Sheridan 1995; *Thorn v. City of Glendale* 1994; Walton 1996), and Divasto and Saxton (1992) wrote an article describing police officers who shoot themselves and create emergencies to gain attention, win acceptance by peers, or escape stress. Nonetheless, this chapter will apply the conceptual framework of FDP to individuals who act out their disorder specifically in health care settings.

Review of Cases

Registered Nurses

The major features of cases involving registered nurses are summarized in Table 9–1.

The nurses in Michigan and Scotland successfully appealed their convictions based on procedural violations (*U.S. v. Narciso* and Perez 1977; *H.M. Advocate v. McTavish* 1974). The Canadian and Maryland cases had produced enough evidence to meet the probable cause standard necessary to arrest and indict the nurses involved; however, neither of these indictments resulted in a conviction, and the epidemiologic study conducted in the Canadian case revealed that the wrong nurse had been arrested. In six cases, as identified in the third column of Table 9–1, the U. S. Centers for Disease Control and Prevention (CDC) conducted epidemiologic studies. The CDC investigations confirmed epidemics associated with the presence of a specific nurse.

Twenty percent of known female serial killers in the United States (Holmes and Holmes 1993) are nurses charged with causing epidemics of patient cardiopulmonary arrest. Interestingly, although 23% of the nurses in Table 9–1 are male, only 5 to 7% of nurses overall are male.

Physicians

Relatively little information is public about most of the serial murder trials involving physicians; thus, the extent of the correlation with the features of FDP is difficult to establish (J. Forrest, unpublished dissertation, 1992). To illustrate, in a Norwegian case, the doctor reportedly tried to use an insanity defense, claiming he had heard voices instructing him to kill his patients. During his crimes, he had used curare (obtained under the pretense that he was going to euthanize his dog) to paralyze his patients into respiratory arrest. Upon confessing, he claimed he was only helping patients who faced a long dying process. However, a psychiatrist witness claimed the physician obtained sexual satisfaction each time he injected a patient and watched him or her die. The jury convicted him of murder, ending a 5-year killing spree that may have involved up to 138 patients (Linedecker and Burt 1990).

Nursing Aides

Table 9–2 summarizes the cases of nurses' aides who have been convicted for murder and assault of patients in their care.

Two cases in which nurses' aides were the perpetrators involved the leader and follower scenario, reminiscent of *folie à deux.* In the 1991 case in Austria, the term *folie à quatre* might apply. Waltraud Wagner, an aide described as both charismatic and highly competent, initiated unauthorized injections. She claimed they were intended to relieve suffering, but the doses were lethal. Eventually, three other aides became involved. They performed a sham "mouth hygiene" procedure that involved holding down the victim's tongue with a tongue depressor, then pouring water into his or her throat to cause drowning (Sereny 1991).

In the other case involving a leader and follower, the aides, both women, were lovers. One, Gwendolyn Graham, allegedly began indoctrinating the other, Katherine Wood, into her scheme of deciding which patients would die. Wood testified that Graham found that killing elderly patients "relieved tension." When Wood told her ex-husband what they were doing, he notified the police (Linedecker and Burt 1990).

In the remaining four cases involving nurses' aides, the aides were men who acted alone. Randy Powers had a history highly suggestive of FDP. He was qualified as a respiratory therapist but had had his license revoked twice. He changed his name, falsified his background, and continued to be hired and fired from a series of jobs in health care facilities.

Table 9–2. Cases involving nurses' aides

Year	Name of perpetrator	Location	Type of unit	Methods
1980	Anders Hansson	Sweden	Geriatrics	Poison (disinfectant)
1984	Randy Powers	California	Hospital	Lidocaine injections
1987	Donald Harvey	Ohio	Hospital	Cyanide in nasogastric tubing
1989	Gwendolyn Graham Katherine Wood	Michigan	Nursing home	Suffocation
1990	Jeffrey Feltner	Florida	Nursing home	Smothering
1991	Waltraud Wagner Stefanija Mayer Maria Gruber Irene Leidolf	Austria	Hospital (three wings)	Injections of insulin and tranquilizers; forcing water into lungs

Powers's first conviction arose after he had initially been hailed as a hero. He had performed cardiopulmonary resuscitation (CPR) on an 11-month-old who became critically ill from an insect bite while in the care of Powers's mother. However, hospital physicians found no sign of an insect bite; instead, there was an injection mark, as well as toxic levels of lidocaine in the child's system. Powers served 2 years of a 5-year sentence for assault. After his release from prison, he changed his name, and was later linked to several other hospital epidemics. Powers was described as meticulous, but he was fired repeatedly for such reasons as not communicating well with patients, stealing patients' personal effects, and appropriating medications. Family members described him as obsessed with becoming a doctor. A few years before he was first arrested, he had won accolades from his neighborhood for adeptly reviving an ill dog (Linedecker and Burt 1990).

Other Caregivers

As noted in Chapter 6, babysitters, foster mothers, and other caregivers have been the perpetrators in some FDP cases (Alexander et al. 1990; *State v. Pankow 1988*; Reed 1992; Richardson 1987; *U.S. v. Woods* 1973; J. Repper, unpublished report, 1994). People in these roles are the logical extensions of mothers who perpetrate. It is less clear in the individual cases of health care professionals—nurses, physicians, and nurses' aides—whether they are compelled by the usual dynamics underlying FDP or whether they are simply serial murderers who perpetrated in the course of employment.

Factitious Disorder by Proxy by Health Professionals

As noted in earlier chapters, DSM-IV defines FDP as "the deliberate production or feigning of physical or psychological signs or symptoms in another person who is under the individual's care" (American Psychiatric Association 1994). DSM-IV limits the motivation for the perpetrator's behavior to the need to assume the sick role by proxy.

Examining the issue more broadly, Meadow (1994) has elaborated on the motivations in the more than 100 cases of FDP he has seen. These motivations have included personal gain, contact with health care providers, publicity, and, occasionally, the attention of an errant partner. More than any other potential motivation, however, the literature is replete with references to the craving for attention that FDP perpetrators exhibit (Feldman and Ford 1994; Schreier and Libow 1993). It is that overriding feature that links the FDP literature with the nurses and other health care professionals accused of serial murder.

Meadow (1994) has stated that the term *Munchausen syndrome by proxy* can be appropriately applied when: 1) illness in the child is invented by a parent or other caregiver; 2) the child is presented for medical assessment and care, usually persistently, often resulting in multiple medical procedures; 3) the perpetrator, at least initially, denies inventing or causing the child's illness; and 4) the signs and symptoms diminish greatly or cease when the child is separated from the perpetrator. If the term *dependent person* is substituted for child, then indeed all of these criteria are met in many of the cases of nurses convicted of serial murder: the nurse invents the patient's illness; the patient typically experiences multiple cardiac arrests and resuscitations; the nurse initially denies any wrongdoing; and the epidemics cease when the culpable nurse is removed from the patient care area.

Serial Murder

A serial killer is defined as someone who murders at least three people over a period longer than 30 days (Holmes and Holmes 1993). Contrary to the vast majority of homicides and assaults, which are acts of violence directed toward specific individuals, the victims of serial murder are generally simply in the wrong place at the wrong time. Serial murder has an underlying compulsive psychological drive, whereas other forms of murder are usually motivated by anger, revenge, money, or jealousy.

A recent study of gender differences in serial murderers (Keeney and Heide 1994) revealed more differences than similarities between males and females on the 14 variables studied. Female serial murderers were more likely to kill victims who were known to them; 43% of their victims were identified as dependents in the custodial care of the murderer. Unlike men, the majority of women used poison (prescribed medications or illicit toxins) as the method of murder. Also in contrast to male serial killers, the women did not stalk their victims, engage in sadistic torture, or engage in violence beyond that needed to cause death. Similarities between male and female serial murderers included race, educational level, employment, and personal histories of abuse during childhood.

Prototypes of FDP

Several of the cases in Table 9–1 exemplify the dynamics of FDP as explicated in Meadow's (1977) and Rosenberg's (1987) work. Genene Jones, the Texas nurse featured in Peter Elkind's book, *The Death Shift*, has been described as having a history of self-injurious behavior, a desperate craving for attention, a need to be in control, and an intense attraction to the world of health care. Jones exhibited the same dualities seen in the FDP mothers—personal feelings of disdain and triumph over the baffled physicians and a coexisting, almost obsequious, dedication to the health care team (Elkind 1989). Schreier and Libow (1993) concur that the case of Genene Jones exemplifies FDP; they included it in their book, *Hurting for Love*. Like Jones, two other convicted nurses have had a documented history of their own self-harm.

The section that follows will describe in greater detail some of the cases listed in Table 9–1 that share many features with classic FDP.

Case 6: Florida, 1984

The Illinois Board of Nursing had previously suspended the license of the nurse convicted in Florida because she had stabbed herself in the vagina with scissors and had required treatment for Munchausen syndrome. Unfortunately, this information did not cross state lines, and she was able to pass the background check and obtain a Florida nursing license. The nursing home administrator who hired her in October 1983 said she was the most conscientious nurse she had ever seen: "She was too good to be true. She came in early for her night shift, she stayed 'til 8 or 9 in the morning charting every linen change, every B.M. each of her patients had. Her nurse's notes were beautiful" (S. Johnson, personal communication, December 1993). Then seven patients died between November 13 and November 23.

On the 23rd, a fire started in the clean linen closet; it was suspected to be arson. On November 26, five more patients died within hours of each other. The next night, the nurse reported being stabbed by a prowler. She was fired from her job after this injury was determined to have been self-inflicted while she was at work.

The State Health Department noted that the death rate for the month at the nursing home had been 25%, a significant increase. When one of the patients who became critically ill during November was successfully treated for unexplained insulin shock (Dahl 1986), a criminal investigation was launched. During the investigation, the CDC epidemiologic study showed that this nurse had been on duty during seven of the shifts on which a terminal event began, and she had been on duty at least 4–8 hours before the onset of four other terminal events (Sacks et al. 1988a).

The former suspension of her license in Illinois was then revealed. Her ex-husband also reported problems with her mental stability; on three occasions she had overdosed their young son with her psychotropic medications. The Department of Family and Children's Services had mandated custody of the 7-year-old to the father because the child had almost died from one overdose (Mayer 1985).

The nurse's medical records showed that, since 1970, she had been hospitalized for a broken arm, gallbladder surgery, ulcers, a hysterectomy, a colostomy, and five other surgeries to treat stomach problems. She also claimed to be waiting for a worker's compensation award for a previous on-the-job injury (Dahl 1986).

Case 4: California, 1981

Another nurse with a history of factitious illness was a male nurse in California in 1981, the oldest perpetrator listed in Table 9–1. Although acquaintances reported that he had always been preoccupied with becoming a doctor, he entered the nursing profession only at the age of 30. A family friend described him as chronically wanting to be a big shot—for example, drawing attention to himself by learning Egyptian healing secrets. He was one of 14 children and reportedly battled several bouts of illness as a child. He was viewed by co-workers as a very competent nurse, but one who also seemed to be on an emotional high when participating in a code. He received a great deal of satisfaction from being in charge and even predicting which patients would die and when (Linedecker and Burt 1990).

The nurse worked at several hospitals and nursing homes until a nursing supervisor insisted that too many unexplained codes were occurring in one of the hospitals. The deaths clustered between 4:00 A.M. and 7:00 A.M., a period during which this nurse was on duty. After bodies were exhumed, lidocaine was found in tissue concentrations too large to have been accidental. Several nurses gave eyewitness accounts of patients dying agonizing deaths with seizures and signs consistent with lidocaine overdose. Syringes with lidocaine, labeled by the nurse, were found in the trash bags of units where he had worked. By the end of the investigation, a staggering 27 deaths of ill, elderly patients were linked to his care. He was found guilty of 12 deaths in two hospitals and sentenced to death. The sentence was upheld on appeal (*People v. Diaz* 1992).

Case 10: New York, 1987

Another case involving a male nurse occurred in New York in 1987. Administrators were alerted when 25 patients died over a 6-week period after experiencing breathing failure. Several other patients survived resuscitative efforts, and one patient reported that the "nurse with a beard had injected something" into his intravenous tubing immediately prior to his experiencing respiratory distress. The rest of the nursing staff found it hard to believe that their well-respected colleague, who was so adept at CPR, could be harming patients.

However, seven of the deaths were deemed suspicious, and eventually the nurse confessed. He stated that his behavior was prompted by his wish to gain respect and attention. He even drew the analogy between his actions and those of a volunteer firefighter who starts a blaze in order to be a hero.

Case 12: Alabama, 1992

A male nurse worked for a registry, or float pool, after being fired from five jobs in Georgia and Alabama. None of his firings involved lack of skill, but rather they occurred either because he had falsified his credentials or time cards or because he had difficulty working with others (*Sheredy et al. v. Twenty Three Medical Facilities* 1992). The Georgia Bureau of Investigation accumulated data on the cardiopulmonary arrests, which clustered during the times this nurse was working at four different hospitals. In addition, patients, after experiencing cardiac arrests and resuscitation, stated that the nurse had injected their intravenous lines immediately prior to the arrest (McDonald 1993). He was ultimately convicted.

Case 13: England, 1993

The 1993 conviction of a nurse in England provides the richest data supporting the link between serial murder by nurses and FDP. The nurse was 23 years old at the time of her conviction for four murders, three attempted murders, and six assaults of pediatric patients. This young woman had grown up, the second of four children, in a small town. She was described by childhood friends as being a good babysitter but also having numerous ill-described ailments. She often had her arm in a sling, and friends began to suspect she was faking the apparent injury.

There were numerous odd incidents during her nursing training, such as feces being found smeared on doors and in the dormitory refrigerator and an inexplicable fire in the kitchen. In addition, her illnesses were exacerbated such that, by the end of her 2 years of training, this nurse had taken 160 sick days with over 50 visits to the infirmary, and 24 to the emergency department. The reasons included a leg injury; two wrist injuries; urinary retention requiring catheterization; appendicitis; and kidney, bladder, and abdominal pain.

By the end of her training, the doctors and physiotherapists were beginning to chart their suspicions of Munchausen syndrome in this woman. She had succeeded in having her normal appendix removed only to return a week later with an infected surgical wound.

Some of her supervisors expressed concern that she needed psychiatric counseling, but there was no follow-through. She had missed so much schooling that she had to repeat 10 weeks in order to qualify as a nurse. Upon completion, she requested assignment to the pediatric ward. After unsuccessfully applying for a 3-year training course to become a pediatric nurse, she was told she needed more experience working with sick children. The head nurse on the unit on which she had trained reluctantly agreed to allow her temporarily to fill their vacancy.

The nurse was hired on February 15, 1991. On the 21st, a child suffered a respiratory arrest on her shift. He was resuscitated, then suffered another and died. Three days later, another child died. There were two arrests of a third child during the nurse's next night shift. The patients' families were very impressed by the care the nurse provided during their children's crises; other nurses also commented on how quickly this new nurse learned to deal with codes.

Within 60 days, however, the pediatric ward had experienced an unprecedented 26 critical incidents, compared with their average of 2 per year. The nurse had insisted on riding in the ambulance to transfer one of the children who had been resuscitated. The family of a twin who had survived an arrest, but which had lost the other twin on the unit, was so taken by the nurse that they asked her to be their surviving daughter's godmother.

Physicians at the pediatric intensive care unit to which five of the children had been transferred were alarmed at the sudden increase in critically ill children, and they requested an investigation. On analysis, a vial of blood from a child who had died showed an elevated insulin level, and the investigation then focused on deliberate causes for the deaths. Evidence of suffocation, air emboli, and toxins were found on postmortem examinations of the children.

The only person present during all 26 incidents was this new nurse. Once arrested, she precipitously lost half her body weight. She was thought to be suffering from anorexia until it emerged that her projectile vomiting was from ingestion of feces. She developed fevers and was so ill during parts of the trial that she could not be in court.

In order to provide the jury with a possible explanation of the motive for these crimes, Dr. Roy Meadow was called as a witness to describe FDP. He recounted his considerable experience with cases of parents who had harmed and even killed their children in ways that he had not thought possible. Asked if it would be difficult to cause deaths on a pediatric ward, he answered no (Davies 1993). The nurse was convicted.

Themes in Nurse-induced Epidemics

Several of the factors that generally underlie FDP emerge during the review of cases of nurse-induced epidemics:

Helpless victims. In all of the cases, the patients who were victimized were physically compromised: they were either critically ill, elderly, or very young. This feature is consistent with the FDP literature, which demonstrates that individuals who are unaware or cannot resist (typically infants and preverbal children) are at greatest risk of being victimized.

Epidemics cluster on the evening and night shifts. This finding is to be expected, since there is more autonomy and less opportunity to be observed by others on the night shifts. This feature correlates with the well-known FDP warning sign that the onset of the child's illness is when only the mother is present and has unobserved time with the child.

Resuscitations. In the cases described, health care personnel were alerted to the likelihood of murder not only by the increased numbers of patient deaths, but by the unprecedented number of patients who experienced successful resuscitation. This finding fits the FDP framework in that most parents with FDP do not intend to kill their children, but intend to bring them to the brink of death to achieve their purpose of creating a medical emergency.

Emotional charge from emergencies. Several of the nurses had been described as getting an emotional high from participating in codes, like mothers with FDP who thrive on the excitement and attention from the medical profession that surrounds the child's critical illnesses.

Described as unusually good nurses. All the nurses studied had the reputations of being excellent, even "model," nurses. They had often been praised for their handling of patient codes. In a similar way, mothers with FDP have characteristically been described as unusually devoted, if not "perfect." Although several of the nurses studied had poor employment records, none of their job losses was because of poor quality nursing. Instead, firings were typically related to their tendency to falsify information, to their personality problems, and to the suspicions prompted by clusters of adverse incidents.

Shock and denial. Other nurses and health care workers at each of the hospitals in which an epidemic occurred experienced shock and disbelief when confronted with evidence that deliberate harm had been perpetrated. In fact, the reluctance of staff to consider this possibility often prolonged the epidemics. This phenomenon mirrors the reaction of pediatric staffs unfamiliar with FDP, who are extremely reluctant to believe that the parent is causing the child's problems.

Denial upon confrontation. Though literature on FDP describes varied reactions of mothers when confronted, the usual reaction is one of denial (Feldman 1994). In the cases described above, whereas there were occasional confessions (with statements such as "I was only trying to help the patients" or "I just needed to appear competent"), confrontation is most notable for continued emphatic denial, even while the nurses are serving jail sentences. The nurses who continue their denial are similar to mothers with FDP who blame hospital staffs for their children's ongoing difficulties. Both convicted nurses and mothers have claimed to be scapegoats for shoddy medical diagnostics or iatrogenic patient incidents.

Personality disorders. Mothers with FDP have been described as exploitive, sadomasochistic, attention-seeking, and wildly erratic in their attitudes toward and relationships with others (Chan et al. 1986). These same descriptors have often been used to apply to the nurses convicted of serial murder.

Recommendations

Physicians, staff members, administrators, and other personnel must be attentive to the possibility, albeit a rare one, that serial murders can occur in their hospitals. Features to consider include the following.

Falsification

As suggested in a number of the cases involving nurses, falsification is often a behavioral manifestation of an underlying personality disorder. Any employee who habitually falsifies information needs to be notified of the seriousness of this behavior and closely monitored, with corresponding documentation produced. Any employee who manufactures crises, including nonmedical ones, is obviously of greatest concern. The British commission that investigated the 1993 case offered several recommendations so stringent that some would not be permissible in the United States:

> 1) We recommend that no candidate for nursing in whom there is evidence of major personality disorder should be employed in the profession; 2) We recommend that, for all those seeking entry to the nursing profession, in addition to routine references the most recent employer or place of study should be asked to provide at least a record of time taken off on grounds of sickness; 3) We recommend that the possibility be reviewed of making available to Occupational Health departments any records of absence through sickness from any institution which an applicant for a nursing post has attended or been employed by. (Her Majesty's Stationary Office 1994)

Epidemics

Routine quality improvement data can reveal clusters of adverse patient outcomes. Early surveillance can pinpoint caregivers or other potential causative factors.

Forensics

It is imperative that good evidence be gathered when a CASK situation is suspected. This information should include epidemiologic data and physical evidence such as syringes, vials of medication, intravenous tubing, and postmortem or postarrest blood studies. Written documentation is also very important. Confessions have sometimes been useful in legal proceedings (Table 9–1).

Conclusion

FDP appears to exist not only within the family but within the occupational setting. A recent study of CASK estimates the prevalence to be one case per million care providers (J. Forrest, unpublished observations, 1992). Improved surveillance and heightened recognition of the phenomenon may show that the prevalence is at least slightly higher than is currently thought.

The paradigm of FDP is very useful in understanding the dynamics of CASK. Meadow's (1993) description of FDP perpetrators is just as applicable to many of the nurses studied: "They tended to be deceitful about many aspects of their personal and past life and to thrive on being the centre of attention or in the midst of crisis."

References

Alexander R, Smith W, Stevenson R: Serial Munchausen syndrome by proxy. Pediatrics 86:581–586, 1990

American Psychiatric Association: Diagnostic and Statistical Manual of Mental Disorders, 4th Edition. Washington, DC, American Psychiatric Association, 1994

Buehler JW, Smith LF, Wallace EM, et al: Unexplained deaths in a children's hospital: an epidemiologic assessment. N Engl J Med 313:211–216, 1985

Chan DA, Salcedo JR, Atkins DM, et al: Munchausen syndrome by proxy: a review and case study. J Pediatr Psychol 11:71–80, 1986

Dahl D: Former nursing home supervisor charged with murder attempt. St. Petersburg Times, March 18, 1986, pp B1, B16

Davies N: Murder on Ward Four. London, Chatto and Windus, 1993

DiVasto P, Saxton G: Munchausen's syndrome in law enforcement. FBI Law Enforcement Bulletin 61:11–14, 1992

Elkind P: The Death Shift: The True Story of Nurse Genene Jones and the Texas Baby Murders. New York, Viking Penguin, 1989

Feldman MD: Denial in Munchausen syndrome by proxy: the consulting psychiatrist's dilemma. Int J Psychiatry Med 24:121–128, 1994

Feldman MD, Ford CV: Patient or Pretender: Inside the Strange World of Factitious Disorders. New York, Wiley, 1994

Foster J: Child killer had been diagnosed in 1986. The Independent, May 19, 1993, p 1

Franks A, Sacks JJ, Smith JD, et al: A cluster of unexplained cardiac arrests in a surgical intensive care unit. Crit Care Med 15:1075–1076, 1987

H.M. Advocate v McTavish, SLT 246-24 (1974)

Her Majesty's Stationary Office: The Allitt Inquiry. London, HMSO, 1994

Holmes RM, Holmes ST: Murder in America. Thousand Oaks, CA, Sage, 1993

Istre GR, Gustafson TL, Baron RC, et al: A mysterious cluster of deaths and cardiopulmonary arrests in a pediatric intensive care unit. N Engl J Med 313:205–211, 1985

Keeney BT, Heide KM: Gender differences in serial murderers. Journal of Interpersonal Violence 9:383–398, 1994

Levin AV, Sheridan MS (eds): Munchausen Syndrome by Proxy: Issues in Diagnosis and Treatment. New York, Lexington, 1995

Linedecker CL, Burt WA: Nurses Who Kill. New York, Windsor Books, 1990

Mayer C: Nurse accused of murder may have poisoned son, ex husband tells court. St. Petersburg Times, May 14, 1985
McDonald RR: The killer nurse. Atlanta Magazine, August 1993, pp 30–38
Meadow R: Munchausen syndrome by proxy: the hinterland of child abuse. Lancet 2:343–345, 1977
Meadow R: False allegations of abuse and Munchausen syndrome by proxy. Arch Dis Child 68:444–447, 1993
Meadow R: Munchausen syndrome by proxy. Journal of Clinical Forensic Medicine 1:121–127, 1994
People v Diaz, 3 Cal 4th 495 (1992)
Reed D: Foster mother suspected in 3 deaths. San Francisco Chronicle, September 24, 1992, pp A1, A17
Repper J: Munchausen syndrome by proxy in health care workers. J Adv Nurs 21:299–304, 1995
Richardson G: Munchausen syndrome by proxy. Am Fam Physician 36:119–123, 1987
Rosenberg DA: Web of deceit: a literature review of Munchausen syndrome by proxy. Child Abuse Negl 11:547–563, 1987
Sacks JJ, Herndon JL, Lieb SH, et al: A cluster of unexplained deaths in a nursing home in Florida. Am J Public Health 78:806–808, 1988a
Sacks JJ, Stroup DF, Will ML, et al: A nurse-associated epidemic of cardiac arrests in an intensive care unit. JAMA 259:689–695, 1988b
Schreier HA, Libow JA: Hurting for Love: Munchausen by Proxy Syndrome. New York, Guilford, 1993
Sereny G: Waltraud's sisterhood of death. The Independent, June 27, 1991
Sheredy et al v Twenty Three Medical Facilities (Fulton County, Ga 1992), Civ Case E-4015 (unreported)
State v Pankow, 144 Wis2d 23 (1988)
Stross JK, Shasby M, Harlan WR: An epidemic of mysterious cardiopulmonary arrests. N Engl J Med 295:1107–1110, 1976
Thorn v City of Glendale, 28 Cal App 4th 1379 (1994)
U.S. v Narciso and Perez, 446 FSupp 252 (ED Mich 1977)
U.S. v Woods, 484 F2d 127 (4th Cir 1973)
Yorker BC: Nurses accused of murder. Am J Nurs 88:1327–1332, 1988
Walton V: Volunteer firefighter arrested in church fire probe. Birmingham News, March 6, 1996, pp 1A–2A
Yorker BC: An analysis of murder charges against nurses. Journal of Nursing Law 1:35–46, 1994

CHAPTER 10

Personal and Interpersonal Toll of Factitious Disorders

Marc D. Feldman, M.D.
Roxenne Smith, M.A.

Very little has been written about the personal and interpersonal consequences of factitious disorders. Reports in the literature usually focus on the objective medical consequences of the disease portrayals. Physical sequelae can indeed range from the removal of healthy organs to the loss of limbs and sometimes even the loss of life itself. The severity of these consequences as well as their stark visibility dramatize the devastating effects of this phenomenon.

However costly these tolls, they tell only half the story. Persons who give their lives to maintaining disease portrayals pay another price in psychosocial terms that are not easily measured but are equally devastating. Just as certainly and profoundly affected are the believers—the family members, friends, and health professionals—who become unwitting participants in the patient's deception.

Increased media attention to the phenomenon of factitious disorder has generated a significant response from patients and the people who have fallen prey to their deceptions. These stories are evidence that the emotional scars left by this disorder cut just as deeply as the physical ones and that the psychosocial toll of factitious disorders may extend over years, if not a lifetime.

Nevertheless, beneath these disquieting tales the message prevails that, with therapy, hope and healing are possible.

Using first person accounts of patients and their caregivers, this chapter examines the personal and interpersonal effects of factitious disorders. A conversational writing style has been deliberately employed in this chapter to reflect more accurately the thoughts and feelings of the individuals who have consented to our use of their stories. Names and identifying details have been altered and the stories edited to ensure anonymity and clarity. The authors' comments within the stories presented are italicized and within brackets.

The Toll of Believing

One of the most disturbing characteristics of patients with factitious disorders is their uncanny ability to perpetuate lies so convincingly that they directly shape the perceptions of those around them. In some cases, the storyteller creates compelling physical signs to support the deceptions. In other cases, the manipulation is accomplished without supporting evidence; instead, the storyteller relies solely on verbal and acting skills. Either way, the stories are generally so engaging and heart wrenching that few people seriously doubt them even when the tales escalate to outlandish proportions.

Case 1

Donna is an articulate, educated, and insightful young woman. Her story provides a remarkably dramatic example of the effect of factitious disorders on caregivers and is a rare case in which the ruse was carried out by a physician. A master manipulator with the expertise to support his deception, the doctor ("Chad") subjected Donna, his fiancée, to more than 2 years of psychological torture. As Donna wrote,

> In February 1991, Chad complained of abdominal pain. He had a biopsy which came back positive for cancer in the lining of his large bowel. He was given radiation every morning and afternoon on a regular basis. I don't remember the exact schedule, but he had black magic marker Xs on his abdomen surrounding

bright red marks from the radiation. Over the next 6 months, the three large bowel tumors shrunk and grew. They were monitored with regular MRIs. Because Chad was a physician, his results were given to him at work over the phone, so I never had the chance to go to the doctor with him. Many times Chad told me how difficult it was to read the MRI because of all the scar tissue.

After about a year, the tumor metastasized again to his small bowel. Around that time he started on an experimental drug which he was able to get through his connections as a doctor. He had marks on his arms from the needles used to infuse the drug. He also began having his stem cells stored so that they could be given back to him if needed at a later date. Sometime around early spring of 1992, Chad's cancer again metastasized, this time to his lung and his liver. I was very angry at the doctors for not being more aggressive with the treatments. After the first metastasis, Chad said he was told that surgery was not an option. I cannot begin to describe the pain and anguish my family and I suffered during these times, the tears that were shed and the prayers that were said. Chad kept my family informed as to his cancer and treatments and, being a physician, he was trusted and believed by all. He would often draw pictures of his tumors to help us understand the situation.

The drug regimen increased, and he became very sick with little appetite. In May of 1992 he went to a nationally known medical center for a second opinion. After a round of consultations, he was told there that he would get the best treatment available. Shortly after, we became engaged and planned a big fall wedding. The extensive treatments continued, but the MRIs showed little change in his tumors and this was extremely upsetting to all of us. Because of the urgency of his situation, his doctors believed that stem cell recovery was his best option. The plans to proceed with surgery were set for early fall, and the wedding had to be canceled.

Since my parents and their friends had purchased nonrefundable airline tickets, I asked Chad for a letter from his doctor so that they could get a refund. He provided me with the letter [*since proved to be a forgery*], which I forwarded to my parents. However, a week before the stem cell procedure was to be performed, Chad had another MRI which showed that the tumors had decreased in size by 50%. In view of this unexpected improvement, the stem cell recovery was canceled.

In July of 1993, while I was out of town, Chad went into cardiac arrest during a treatment and had to be shocked back to life. When I returned, he had two burn marks on either side of his heart from the paddle marks used to shock him. Around this time he also began bleeding from his colon because one of the tumors was eating into an artery. I gave him sanitary napkins to wear. He spent many weekend days in bed, and I saw the bloody napkins in the trash. I was totally committed to him during this time and was prepared to stay with him until the end, whether that be his recovery or his death. As a young woman, I cannot tell you how devastating this was for me, to watch my future husband slowly die.

In the fall of 1993, he became extremely depressed, and we frequently discussed his stopping the treatments because they were destroying his quality of life. We cried together numerous times, and I told him he had to be strong and continue. At the end of September, he told me had considered suicide. One night, in a state of severe depression, he called his brother. His brother, who was also a physician, immediately came for him and took him to a psychiatric center. Chad called sobbing from the center and told me they were going to admit him. I asked to speak with his brother, whom I had never met. A few seconds later, this cold voice came on the line. His brother made me feel as if I had failed to take care of Chad. He said that he and the doctors decided that Chad could call me only once a day. He would not tell me where they were. For the next 5 days, I continued to speak with both Chad and his brother by phone.

I did not trust his brother and had a growing suspicion that something was wrong. I went to the library and looked up his brother in a directory of physicians. Then I looked up Chad. Piecing the facts together, I learned then that Chad had lied about his age, claiming to be 9 years younger than he actually was. More importantly, when I used the number in the directory to place a phone call to his brother, I learned that he had been out of the country for some time and that he had not yet returned. I suddenly realized that the person I had been speaking with for the past 5 days, and whom I believed to be Chad's brother, was in fact Chad himself. I shudder at the thought of how he could be sobbing one minute and speaking to me in a cold dispassionate voice the next. I became frightened that Chad would come after me and hurt me, knowing now how mean he could be.

Though I was dumbstruck, I complied with Chad's request that I retrieve his messages from work. I called one of Chad's

> co-workers to see when I could pick the messages up and discovered that she was at a scientific meeting in Ontario. The next day I called the convention center in Ontario to try and locate his co-worker. Something also made me ask if "Chad Bentley" was registered. When the operator said "One minute, I'll connect you," I was flabbergasted. Chad was in Ontario, not a local psychiatric hospital. I tried to call him all night, but he was not in the hotel room. Early the next morning he called and continued to tell me how he was opening up with the mental health counselors. I played along and then called him back at the hotel an hour later. He hung up on me. I finally reached his co-worker, who answered my many questions about Chad's previous behavior. I learned that Chad had not missed work, was always in his office, and had not shown any signs of illness. She said that, quite to the contrary, he had just been playing golf in Ontario and seemed to be having a great time.
>
> That night Chad called me and tried to continue the charade even though I had discovered his lies. After several minutes he made a number of startling confessions: he had faked the cancer, was indeed 9 years older than he had claimed, and was still married. Then he begged my forgiveness. For 2 years, my family and I had been manipulated for Chad's own amusement into believing he was dying a horrible death. This man has a mental sickness beyond comprehension, and I've had no contact with him since. But I've learned that the day after his "confession" to me, he showed up at work wearing an eye patch, and for the last year, he's been telling co-workers that he has ocular cancer. He's moved on to a new audience.

Chad's symptoms, so cruelly and cleverly executed, devastated his devoted fiancee. So convincing were his disease forgeries that for 2 years Donna's perceptions and emotions were shaped by falsehoods. Unlike most patients with factitious disorders, Chad's motives seem to have stemmed not only from a desire for sympathy but also entailed an ample degree of gratuitous, even sadistic, lying and manipulation.

Not all patients build their deceptions on apparent physical evidence, such as Chad did when he created marks and burns on his skin and soaked gauze pads with blood. Some rely solely on the power of the story. Even when evidence is absent or contradictory, the deceptions often gain momentum nevertheless, and more people are drawn in.

Case 2

Anna's case illustrates the power of factitial lies. Both child protection and law enforcement interdiction were mobilized against two parents as a result of spurious allegations of physical and sexual abuse. Anna's mother wrote, shortly after Anna had turned 12,

> Last September, I was approached by Child Protective Services [CPS] and told that my daughter, Anna, had confided in a camp counselor that her father had been sexually molesting her through the years. I had never even considered that this could be happening; I thought the charge was ridiculous. Although I still felt fairly sure her stories were not true, by the time I had been interrogated by the child protection workers, I had to open my mind to the possibility. I tried to follow the professionals' advice, and, although my husband was devastated and totally denied ever having harmed my daughter, she and I moved out of the house. [*Anna leveled accusations that predictably mobilized the immediate attention of authorities. Even her mother began to entertain the possibility of abuse despite having initially considered the story to be ridiculous. These accusations produced the disintegration of Anna's family life.*]
>
> Everyone kept telling me I had to back up Anna completely or she would be terribly damaged. I honestly tried. Over time, Anna's school had become very involved in the entire situation, and she was getting lots of attention as a child who was apparently abused. But as time went on, her stories just didn't make sense. Still, it seemed that I was the only one, besides my husband, who cared that there were inconsistencies.
>
> What happened next made me see the light. Anna began injuring herself and then accusing me of physical abuse. Since I had had no idea that this story-telling was going on, it was a major shock when I suddenly found myself on the hot seat. She produced marks on herself and said that I had burned her. She applied "bruises" with makeup. She would suddenly feign being hysterical and run to a neighbor's house, claiming I was beating her, and I was charged with abuse. Anna would sometimes confess to doctors that I was not really harming her, but then she would switch back to the accusations involving my husband and they would focus on that.
>
> The first contact my husband was allowed to have with Anna came months later. Upon the recommendation of the child protective agency, I made sure they were never alone with each

> other. I thought the visit had been a success, but 2 days later, CPS called to say that Anna's father had forced her to have sexual intercourse with him during their time together. Her details were absolutely convincing, so believable that I actually followed their advice and had her examined by an expert in sexual abuse. There was no evidence of penetration.
>
> The months have passed, and we've been through several more crises. Anna now says that none of it was true and she has no idea why she does these things. Luckily, charges have been dropped against me and my husband. It is incredible that a child who is otherwise sweet could do the things she has.

Case 3

A central motive in many cases of factitious victimization is the search for nurturance by individuals who have felt unable to obtain it in more adaptive ways. The allegation by a child of physical assault and rape is particularly charged with emotion, and generally our legal and child protective systems support the notion that children do not lie about abuse. Stemming from a desire to protect the vulnerable, such precautions have been instrumental in removing children from abusive situations; however, they have also at times been hastily employed when there is abundant evidence to the contrary. The following letter was received from a prison inmate:

> My life was changed forever when a child falsely accused me of sexual molestation last year. Although the child named me, I am not the perpetrator and, as time passes, there is increasing doubt that any molestation even occurred. I recognize that the state is obligated to pursue such cases, but my trial is to be held soon. I am bewildered and frightened, and I have few family members left able to help me.

In both cases cited previously, the lives of the accused hinged on accusations for which no genuine evidence existed. In Anna's case, her dramatic ruses eventually exposed her false claims of abuse; yet, when it came to accusations against her father, it was immediately his character, not hers, that was called into question. Regardless of the patient's age or circumstance, the trust elicited by patients with factitious disorder is quite typical. These patients are masterful at manipulating events to match their stories, so that even as a deception begins to unravel, the lie is being continuously retooled to keep the believer engaged.

When the inconsistencies become too great to ignore, caregivers, including medical professionals, often experience a clinical dilemma—to confront or not to confront. The decision to confront may be an emotional Catch-22. If the story of physical or psychological woe turns out to be true and the caregiver has doubted it, he or she bears responsibility for increasing the individual's anguish. However, if the caregiver ignores the evidence and chooses to believe what may be a lie, he or she has abetted the patient in an illness that is both physically and psychologically dangerous.

A cruel irony exists for all believers who have truly cared for the deceiver. In unveiling a lie, the caregiver's deepest hopes are fulfilled: a lover's health is suddenly restored, or the rape of a beloved daughter never happened. However, when such a burden is suddenly exposed as specious it may irreparably damage the relationship.

The Toll on the Other Parent

Of the various presentations of factitious disorder, factitious disorder by proxy (FDP) has received the bulk of recent media attention. Generally, this coverage centers on the most common variant: mothers who are accused of abusing or murdering their children in order to assume the sick role indirectly. In cases in which the mother maintains that she is innocent of harming her child, she may be presented as the victim of outrageous lies that may cause the unjust loss of her parental rights. In cases in which FDP is acknowledged, she may be portrayed again as a victim, this time of an acknowledged mental disorder against which she is helpless. Whereas the affected children are properly viewed as the most in need of attention and protection, the fathers in many ways are the forgotten victims of FDP, and their stories are seldom heard. There are two reasons for the dearth of information from and about fathers. First, fathers are as unlikely as medical and legal professionals to associate the mother with the child's unexplained illnesses or death. Second, even when FDP has been implicated in child abuse cases, the father is likely to ally himself with the mother against the authorities (Zitelli et al. 1987). Ray's case provides a unique perspective on the toll taken by FDP on fathers who love their children and will risk a great deal to protect them.

Case 4

Ray's story began months before the birth of his first child. His seemingly idyllic marriage to the woman he was "crazy about" suddenly took a turn when she discovered she was pregnant. Though they had been married only 2 months earlier, his new bride suddenly rejected any form of intimacy and showed increasing aggression toward him. Ray provides the following account:

> Once Janet found out she was pregnant, her attitude changed immediately. She would not eat or sleep with me. She would get mad if I even kissed her on the cheek. We talked and it was as if her aloofness were all my fault. Suddenly I was the husband from hell. I couldn't understand what was going on. I just thought it was because she was pregnant.
>
> Then I thought that maybe my reaction to her pregnancy was not what she was looking for. My reaction had been, "Oh my goodness. You're pregnant." We had just gotten married and bought this house. I was the only one working. I had just changed jobs and my insurance hadn't kicked in and I was looking at some big bills. It was the financial concern that first came to my mind. And that was wrong. I admit that. I pressed for answers, but I never had any suspicion that she was a very sick person. As the weeks passed, things got worse and worse. She stayed in her room. She barely spoke to me. I was determined to understand the problem and I tried to get her to talk about it. One day we were upstairs in the bedroom having a heated discussion about the way things were going. When I got up to leave, she followed me to the top of the stairs and then pushed me hard. I fell to the bottom. I was extremely shaken, but essentially unhurt.
>
> Not long after this happened, I came home from work one day and all her stuff was gone. There was no note. I was shocked and hurt and I felt just terrible. I discovered that she had drained the checking and savings accounts and, soon after, I received notice that she was suing for divorce.
>
> At our first court hearing I was instructed to pay all her medical expenses. I told myself that this was my child too, so I had no problem bearing the cost, but I had no idea how much cost

I would ultimately bear. During her pregnancy she ran up a bill of nearly $8,000 for seven emergency room visits. These expenses were in addition to the set fee for regular prenatal care and delivery. I had no contact with her at all during her pregnancy except through the attorneys. I just kept paying the bills, figuring that the care was necessary.

In my county, divorce is not granted in cases of pregnancy until after the child is born. Nine days after my son was born, Janet called me and it nearly knocked me out because I did not think I would hear from her again. She told me my son was sick and in the hospital. I had not yet seen my child. I was both elated at the news of his birth and sick to death that something was wrong. I drove to the hospital with my heart in my throat. [*This was the first of three hospital admissions for alleged apnea, although the mother was the only one to witness these spells. Apnea is among the most common presenting complaints in FDP* (Rosenberg 1987).]

When I saw my son for the first time, I cannot tell you how I felt. He was so small. He had just had a spinal tap and he looked so miserable. For the next 10 days, he remained in the hospital, and the doctors put him through every test known to man, but couldn't find anything wrong with him. [*Characteristically of FDP mothers, Janet was extremely willing to have her child undergo numerous tests and procedures, and in fact expressed irritation that more tests were not being performed.*] They thought his problem might be due to an infection, but they found no infection. Then they thought it had something to do with the shape of his heart; there was nothing wrong with his heart. They tested his blood; everything checked normal. They did sleep studies on him, and they performed an amazing number of other tests. Finally, they sent him home.

About 2 weeks later, my son was back in the hospital. He remained in intensive care hooked up to monitors and undergoing another round of tests. No abnormalities were discovered, and eventually he was sent home again. Around this time I happened to see a TV show on Munchausen syndrome by proxy and it struck a tremendous chord with me. Before this, I had not made a connection between Janet's E.R. visits during her pregnancy and my son's E.R. visits now. I couldn't stop thinking about this.

When the next call came telling me that my son was once again in the hospital, I was ready to voice my suspicions. This was his third hospitalization. At 3 months of age, he had spent most of his life in the hospital. I'll never forget: I walked in to see him and they had this gauze helmet on my son and he looked totally miserable. I made him a promise. I said "Son, I'm going to take care of you." I was determined that something was going to be done.

There was a young psychiatrist on staff who was assigned to my son's case, and she asked me if there might be any family history that could be causing my son's problem. I just came right out with it. I told her that I thought my wife was causing the repeated apneas. She reminded me that my wife had been a doting mother. "She is up here every day. She never leaves his side," the doctor said. [*FDP mothers are characteristically doting and attentive and are actively engaged in their child's care. This is one reason why FDP is underrecognized.*] But I told her that every time my son had gotten sick, he had been alone with his mother. I asked her to please look into it.

Soon after, I received word that my son was going to be released. I was frantic. I called the psychiatrist and asked her to please reconsider until my suspicions had been more thoroughly investigated. She told me that she was not at liberty just yet to discuss with me what was going on, but that I should trust her. I had no idea what to think. I was going berserk.

Within a half hour I learned that the state had filed a complaint against Janet and had assumed custody of my son. My attorney asked me if I wanted custody. I told him I wanted this child more than anything in the world.

For 1 week my son remained in foster care while the Department of Human Resources did a study on my fitness as a parent. I passed with flying colors and was granted temporary custody for 6 months. My son was placed on a home apnea monitor and there was never a problem of any kind the whole time I had him.

After 6 months, I went back to court to obtain permanent custody. Janet's attorney was brilliant in his case presentation. Things did not look good for my son and me. [*The judge viewed it as counterintuitive that an apparently loving mother could produce an illness in her child, that induced apnea could have eluded detection in the past, and that an allegedly abusive mother would lack a history of overt criminal behavior.*] I was so nervous that during this period I would wake up in the middle of the night scared to death, thinking, "He's not here." It was like a bad dream. I thought, "What will I do if they take him from me?" But I had made a promise to my son to take care of him and I was prepared to leave the country if it came to that.

When the state's deputy coroner was called in, things began turning around for us. The deputy coroner began questioning

> Janet about her previous child. [*As Ray had also informed the hospital staff at the time of his frantic call to them, Janet's child from a previous marriage had died at age 2 after being treated for recurrent breathing problems and seizures of unexplained etiology. This child's medical history had included 4 hospitalizations and 10 emergency room visits.*] The state also brought in an expert witness on Munchausen syndrome by proxy. The presence of these two witnesses resulted in my ex-wife's sudden decision to relinquish all custody rights.

One year later, Ray's son is a thriving, healthy child. He has had no further episodes of apnea or respiratory problems of any kind while under his father's care.

The Toll on Professional Caregivers

The psychological state behind self-induced or feigned illnesses is difficult for most people to understand. It is hard enough to accept that a person is engaging in self-harm; the fact that he or she is seeking emotional gratification through such behavior predictably elicits little sympathy. The deceit underlying the disease forgery only contributes to this unsympathetic attitude, which may tacitly communicate, "Never darken my door again" (Nicholson and Roberts 1994). No one likes to feel like a fool. Professional caregivers have admitted to finding factitious patients reprehensible, and mental health professionals are no less immune to such feelings of intolerance and even disgust. Though the term *Munchausen syndrome* (Asher 1951) actually applies only to the most intractable subset of patients with factitious disorder (Feldman and Ford 1994), at times it is misapplied pejoratively to dismiss treatment efforts directed toward any patient who has feigned or manufactured an illness, even as an isolated occurrence. Thus, once a deception has been exposed, the patient, if he or she is willing to access help, may have a difficult time finding a therapist with whom an alliance can be forged (Feldman and Feldman 1995).

Similarly, professional caregivers who have been duped by a factitial illness may receive marginal or no support from other professionals. They may be derided for what is viewed as their "rescue fantasies," "delusions of grandeur" in hoping to be able to help (Willenberg 1994), or general lack of professional judgment.

Case 5

Colleen, a college advisor who was duped by a student who made repeated false claims of illness, explains how she was treated when the deception was exposed:

> I had worked tirelessly to obtain for this student the help she appeared so desperately to need. I put in many extra hours and admit to having become too involved. In hindsight this is easy to recognize; but at the time, I felt compelled by simple human compassion to see this young woman through what, to all appearances, was a valiant struggle against cancer. Anything else would have seemed harsh and unfeeling.
>
> My supervisor was aware of the extra time I was expending. She applauded my effort and offered her support and encouragement, checking frequently on my progress with the student. When the deception was revealed, however, my extra effort was suddenly labeled as inappropriate involvement. This supervisor insisted that I be issued a written reprimand.
>
> If I had any question about my own professionalism in this situation (and I had plenty), in my mind all doubts were now dispelled. I now had a signed statement in my file that verified that I had indeed acted unprofessionally. As long as the student's deception worked, I was perceived as a good and valuable worker. When the deception was revealed, I was perceived as lacking professionalism. In truth, it was easier for me to forgive the student than it was the body politic that operated under such a double standard. I felt betrayed on two counts. [*When a deception is disclosed, the caregiver is often overwhelmed emotionally. Accepting the evidence is often the most difficult task a professional helper faces.*]
>
> I resisted all evidence that she might be lying. I did not want to believe that all my efforts to help her, my sleepless nights, my unmitigated anxiety over her well-being had been based on a lie. I did not want to feel how furious I actually was with her. And I was shamed by the fact that I had not helped my client at all but had in fact enabled her in her illness. I felt I should have known better. [*Once a deception is acknowledged, feelings of anger and guilt are equally common. Often these feelings are of such intensity that health care professionals may themselves need professional help in processing their feelings. To help the helper, therapists need an understanding of factitious disorders and the profound impact of factitious deception. To date, the lack of awareness surrounding factitious disorders places few therapists in the field who can fully respond to the unique emotional*

needs of deceived helpers. Nevertheless, Colleen was able to gain a great deal of insight from working with a therapist, and she attributes her emotional healing to therapeutic intervention.]

I was totally devastated by my experience. Three months after the event, I was still suffering from insomnia and found no relief at all from my feelings of guilt, anxiety, and depression. I finally decided to ask for help. The therapist helped me in translating my guilt and depression more appropriately into anger. She also provided the compassion and understanding that was lacking in my work environment. It was a great relief to have someone in my corner.

Much later, when I read an article about factitious disorder, I contacted my therapist. She was amazed to learn that my experience had been the result of a diagnosable disorder; she had never heard the term before. Just knowing about factitious disorder, she said, could have been very comforting to me at the time, and she expressed her regret over not having been able to help me in that way.

This story highlights not only the reaction of caregivers but also the importance of professional education about all of the forms of factitious disorders. For example, in a study by Blix and Brack (1988), 70% of a group of staff nurses felt both personally and professionally unprepared to respond to a case of FDP uncovered in their hospital. After detection, nearly 40% of them reported that they had become less trusting of parents and guardians in general. Inservices by a psychiatric liaison nurse have been proposed as a remedy for such profound reactions (Miller and Cabeza-Stradi 1994).

Miller and Cabeza-Stradi (1994) have written specifically about the toll on nurses forced suddenly to confront the issue of Munchausen syndrome. In this report, a patient claiming to be a critical care nurse recounted numerous surgeries as a result of accidents, muggings, and other misfortunes. She readily elicited empathy from the staff, and she had extensive bleeding and hematuria with clots. Although no organic explanation for the bleeding was identified, a nephrectomy (her second) was performed. While preparing her room for her return from surgery, however, one nurse inadvertently discovered concealed needles, syringes, and two anticlotting medications (urokinase and streptokinase), which the patient could easily have injected into her

Hickman catheter to induce the bleeding. The discovery of the deception led to waves of anger among the staff. This encounter was, for all the nurses, their first experience with factitious disorders. Inservices for the nurses were held to address their professional responsibilities to the patient, who remained on the ward. Some nurses indicated that they preferred not to care for this particular patient and asked for alternate assignments.

Support groups were offered as well to focus on the overwhelming feelings of the staff. It proved important for support group members to find similarities and differences in their feelings in order to master them. Many members found it hard to move past the initial phase of anger. Nonetheless, the effort continued avidly, and ultimately with good results, since nurses who are not able to deal effectively with the feelings of betrayal may be affected adversely in their careers (Blix and Brack 1988).

Living With the Specter

Factitious disorders deeply influence both patients and their families. Healing cannot begin until the deception is exposed; but long after a deception ends, disturbing elements of factitious disorder may remain. The task of finding new outlets for satisfying one's deep emotional needs is indeed a challenging one, and the impulse to feign illness may continue for years. Thus, neither patients nor their families easily emerge from the shadow of this troubling disorder. Nevertheless, the hope of recovery is offered in the stories of patients who have overcome the greatest barrier of all, confronting the real illness—the factitious disorder—head on.

Abe's case offers a look at the emotional needs driving the impulse to fake an illness. It also sheds light on how factitious behaviors, even after they have ceased, continue to impact a patient's life.

Case 6

By age 16, Abe had devoted 3 years of his life to faking asthma attacks, a rare type of factitious ailment (Baker and Major 1994). As is often the case among patients with factitious disorders, Abe's feigning of illness began after he was hospitalized for an authentic physical problem. According to Abe,

When I was discharged from the hospital, everyone kept wanting to know how I was feeling and what they could do for me. My mother came running home from work and my dad was even concerned about me. I have to say, it was a pretty incredible feeling. I truly felt loved.

But after a while it seemed like it never happened, and life went back to normal around here. Could I let that happen? Could I go from getting all the attention and love anyone could ever need or want to being just plain Abe? I decided I needed another wheezing episode just to make people a little nervous. I went to the school nurse, and when she listened to my chest, this time I "induced" a wheeze; that is, I made a high pitched stridor that radiated to the lungs and sounded like a wheeze. The doc was called, and I went to the E.R. Mom came home from work and Dad was concerned all over again. Wow! This attention was great! [*Abe's relationship with his father had always been strained. Throughout his life he believed himself to be a vast disappointment to his father. For the first time, Abe felt as if he were receiving from his father the validation that he so greatly desired.*]

In the next month I would escalate the symptoms over and over again and the ambulance would come to my house at least four times a week. The odd thing is that at this point, the impulse to fake was stronger than any impulse I had ever felt before. [*As the disorder progresses, the impulse to fake or create signs and symptoms can become so strong that it completely overpowers the natural human impulse toward self-protection.*] Also, I saw my mom and dad suffering, and as much as it hurt me on the one hand, I enjoyed it on the other. I mean this was great—revenge and attention.

I was eventually sent away to a top respiratory hospital where I became an inpatient for 6 weeks. During that time I faked many, many attacks. I fooled them too. Now the stakes were even higher. It was more than just the attention and revenge; it was pulling one over on those "stupid" doctors. It was the anger that I could never express to my dad displaced onto the entire medical profession.

When I was discharged, I was sent home with the diagnosis of mild bronchial asthma. Little did I know that I truly did have asthma, and that by not taking my medication (which I was flushing down the toilet) I was making my real asthma worse. After 10 or 20 new doctors, 100 E.R. visits, 10 hospital admissions for status asthmaticus, countless doses of intravenous steroids, and hundreds of epinephrine injections, I was sent back for reevaluation. That's when the truth would come out.

> The process of recovery from 3 years of factitious disorder has been hard. First, I would have to determine how much of my asthma was real and how much was my making it up. I had lost track of that. Then I would have to deal with the side effects that I had from the steroids, like osteoporosis and Cushing's syndrome. Three years of my life had been controlled by this impulse to fake. I had no social life. I was on home study from school. Every thought and breath was centered on my illness. Before this whole mess started clearing up, I would be in two psychiatric institutions and attempt suicide numerous times. I figured if I couldn't get the same degree of attention and love I had when I was "sick," I just wanted to die. I didn't think that I could deal with the humiliation of coming back into my life and having to tell people I faked my illness.

Although the exposure of Abe's ruse caused him to fear the humiliation he would face in reentering the world, it was also his first hope for stopping the behavior. When a deception begins to unravel, most patients will, at least initially, ply their best tactical strategies to keep the ruse going and thereby maintain the interest of those around them. Still, however stressful exposure may be, some patients admit ultimately to wanting to be caught. Some of these patients relish disclosure because it is only in this way that their doctors will realize that, even as highly educated professionals, they have been "outsmarted" and "defeated" by the patient. Other patients with factitious disorder, tired of the endless effort involved in maintaining a deception and aware that their behaviors are abnormal and/or life-threatening, try authentically to gain an understanding of their actions. For these people, a lie exposed offers the hope of successful treatment.

Patients who do consent to therapy often feel dubious about their future, shifting alternately between the hope of recovery and the fear of returning to their former ways. Denise's story in the following case illuminates the painful interplay between these two psychological states.

Case 7

> I became masterful at feigning illness. What began as a relatively innocent set of symptoms soon evolved into an elaborate scheme that included several induced cases of peritonitis, blood stream

infections, false blindness, paralysis, and other conditions. These were coupled with many incidents of self-mutilation that were always referred to as accidents. For 2 years I was diagnosed as having fever of unknown origin. I believe that at final count I had had 25 major surgeries. The scars I bear from head to toe serve as constant reminders of this turbulent period of my life.

When I was 18, this tangled web I had woven was getting old. I was tired of the game and came to the realization that no one was going to catch me. If there was to be a change, it would have to come from within. I committed myself to a state hospital. I took this action despite the heated protest of my family. I continued to feign some illnesses but concentrated more on self-mutilation, such as cutting my forearms. In retrospect, I realize that my desire to end the fraud did not simultaneously equip me to cope with life. Until I learned new skills, I had to continue on a path I wanted so desperately to avoid.

Patients who sincerely want to end their behaviors express a pained bewilderment over their inability to stop. Their actions are incomprehensible to them. Some patients openly admit to being repulsed by their own behaviors but cannot find a way to end them. In the following letter, the patient's conflict is evident. Like Denise's, Sally's account in the following case reflects her inner battle; underlying her troubled state is a cry for help.

Case 8

Ever since I was in middle school, I've been telling stories or lies. They aren't true at all, but I still like making them up. I've been trying to stop, but nothing works. I'm still doing this stupid stuff. I go to a psychologist and see a social worker. I've been with the psychologist for 4 years now. Even though sometimes I feel like I'm moving forward, overall I am still stuck. Why am I like this? It's confusing to me.

The hope and fear depicted in these accounts are not unique to the patient with factitious disorder. If patients themselves swing precariously between hope for recovery and fear of relapse, family members also experience the same alternating feelings. Because factitious disorders can present in the young, and sometimes the very young, parents understandably search and hope for the best possible outcome, even in the worst of circumstances.

In the case of Anna, whose allegations of physical and sexual abuse were described earlier, her mother poignantly expresses the array of feelings she has toward her daughter:

> Anna is on medication and is doing well currently, but since we still don't know what caused all this in the first place I can't feel confident it won't resurface. The last psychiatrist that treated her in the hospital said she felt Anna was hopeless and we needed to put her somewhere for our safety as well as hers. Needless to say, I didn't continue with her.
>
> As Anna left for her first day of junior high school today, she appeared to be a happy, well-adjusted 12-year-old. I only wish I could believe it. I love my daughter very much and wish her creative talents could be steered in the right direction.

In time, some families find they can no longer sustain the psychological tensions of living amid a tangle of fact and fantasy, and they choose to end their relationship with the patient. For example, parents, bereft of emotional and even financial resources, may find that they have to cut their own child out of their lives as their only means of survival.

As factitious disorders receive increased notice through mass media exposure, a new picture is emerging that is helping to counter tacit convictions of therapeutic nihilism among mental health professionals. Like Abe, several patients with factitious disorders have come forward to disclose their long-held secrets and to serve as testimonials to the healing effect of education and therapy. The words of Denise powerfully convey the possibility of recovery offered through these interventions. She writes,

> I am in therapy at this time and continue to work diligently to better understand my motives and needs which caused me to take such drastic measures. As I slowly uncover the many abuses to which I was subjected in childhood, my subsequent behaviors are more understandable, and indeed my past actions were reasonable. They served their purpose well by removing me from a destructive situation and placing me in one in which there was safety and nurturing. The tragedy is that I paid such a high price for safety.
>
> When I viewed a TV segment on factitious disorder, I experienced a freedom which was indescribable. It was as though I was seeing and hearing my own story. For the first time I felt affirmed

in the realization that I was not the only person who had harmed my body in such drastic ways. Just having a name for my experience offered incredible affirmation. [*This statement is heard again and again from both patients and their families and caregivers. As in the cases of other mental disorders, having a name for the disordered behavior offers almost immediate comfort. Embodied in the nomenclature is the realization that one has not been alone in this experience.*]

The door has been opened for me to claim my actions and accept them. I have spent inordinate energy keeping this door shut, and believe me, the idea that it can be opened and its contents explored can be likened to getting a whole new lease on life.

I would gamble to say that most people caught in this downward spiral would like to get out of it if only they knew how and were certain that they could find love in more acceptable ways. Just the knowledge that one is not alone, that the experience is understood, and that changes are possible offers so much promise for those who are trapped. The more the word is spread, the greater the likelihood of Cinderella stories. It is possible to get out of the trap. I know. I've done it.

References

Asher R: Munchausen syndrome. Lancet 1:339–341, 1951

Baker CE, Major E: Munchausen's syndrome. A case presenting as asthma requiring ventilation. Anaesthesia 49:1050–1051, 1994

Blix S, Brack G: The effects of a suspected case of Munchausen's syndrome by proxy on a pediatric nursing staff. Gen Hosp Psychiatry 11:402–409, 1988

Feldman MD, Feldman JM: Tangled in the web: countertransference in the therapy of factitious disorders. Int J Psychiatry Med 25:379–389, 1995

Feldman MD, Ford CV: Patient or Pretender: Inside the Strange World of Factitious Disorders. New York, Wiley, 1994, pp 23–25

Miller M, Cabeza-Stradi S: Addiction to surgery: a nursing dilemma. Crit Care Nurse 14:44–48, 1994

Nicholson SD, Roberts GA: Patients who (need to) tell stories. Br J Hosp Med 51:546–549, 1994

Rosenberg DA: Web of deceit: a literature review of Munchausen syndrome by proxy. Child Abuse Negl 11:547–563, 1987

Willenberg H: Countertransference in factitious disorder. Psychother Psychosom 62:129–134, 1994

Zitelli BJ, Seltman MF, Shannon RM: Munchausen's syndrome by proxy and its professional participants. Am J Dis Child 141:1099–1102, 1987

CHAPTER 11

Management of Factitious Disorders

Stuart J. Eisendrath, M.D.
Adriana Feder, M.D.

In this chapter, the authors focus on treatment approaches for factitious physical and psychological disorders. Because factitious physical disorders have been best studied, their treatment will be discussed first and at greater length. Interventions and management strategies for factitious disorder by proxy are discussed elsewhere in this volume.

Factitious Physical Disorders

Beginning with Asher's (1951) description of the Munchausen syndrome, physicians have tried to develop a systematic approach to managing factitious physical disorders. Birch (1951) urged the formation of a registry to identify and track factitious physical disorder cases. Although never actually implemented, the registry was conceptualized with the goal of alerting physicians and preventing iatrogenic complications as patients traveled from one city to another. Requests for similar registries have continued to arise intermittently since then (Ifudu et al. 1992). Ethical and legal restrictions, however, have precluded this approach in the United States (see Chapter 4).

Growing awareness of the economic costs of factitious disorders have added urgency to finding effective interventions. Cohen et al. (1985) have identified the high costs of failing to identify and treat psychiatric disorders that occur in the medical setting. Powell and Boast (1993) reported the "Million Dollar Man" with factitious physical disorder in Great Britain. Reports in the United States similarly indicate that costs can be enormous (Feldman 1994) and easily exceed one million dollars when life-threatening factitious disorders are produced (Bright, unpublished observations).

In the following sections, we examine several strategies that have been developed to treat factitious physical disorders. Although no reports have yet been published concerning actual cost savings from these strategies, there is great potential for conservation of medical resources.

Pharmacotherapy

Some clinicians have found that medication is of value for selected patients with factitious physical disorder. Fras and Coughlin (1971) noted that one patient whom they treated benefited from a phenothiazine for psychotic episodes. Earle and Folks (1986) suggested that many patients with factitious physical disorders have borderline personality disorders and may benefit from the use of antipsychotic medication during brief periods of psychosis and disorganization. These recommendations are similar to those of Van Moffaert (1989), who advocated antipsychotic medications for self-mutilating patients.

Some clinicians have considered factitious physical disorders, particularly when connected with multiple surgical procedures, to be parasuicidal behaviors and associated with depressive syndromes (Menninger 1934). Earle and Folks (1986) treated a patient for whom depression appeared prominent, and an antidepressant was effective in improving mood and diminishing factitious behavior. Other authors (Geracioti et al. 1987; Plassmann 1994a) have suggested that object loss may activate episodes of factitious disorder, strengthening the rationale for treating depression. More recently, there has been an abundance of literature describing various conditions as part of the obsessive-compulsive disorders spectrum (McElroy et al. 1994; Rasmussen 1994). In some cases of factitious physical disorder, the behavior may have compulsive qualities. It is tempting to speculate that these individuals may be responsive to the selective serotonin reuptake inhibitors that have been so successful in obsessive-compulsive disorders. However, there have been no systematic pharmacologic trials for the factitious disorders. Undoubtedly, this deficit has been related to the difficulty of engaging many of these patients in ongoing psychiatric treatment.

Despite these prospects, patients with factitious physical disorders infrequently present with another overarching Axis I disorder such as major depression that readily responds to medication trials (Folks and Houck 1993). In addition, many patients with factitious physical disorders will be reluctant to try explicitly psychiatric medications, particularly in the early stages of treatment; because these patients do not admit to the factitious nature of their ailments, psychotropic medication is resisted. Thus, the primary approach to treatment of factitious physical disorders rests with psychological interventions.

Psychotherapeutic Strategies

Confrontational Approaches

Early attempts to manage factitious physical disorders typically involved confronting the patient with evidence of the factitious behavior. For example, laboratory findings disclosing the factitious etiology might be brought to the patient's room. The confrontation was often an angry one in which the physician essentially indicted the patient with the evidence. Because this approach was generally not effective in changing the patient's behavior, Hollender and Hersh (1970) developed a creative refinement that attempted to avoid any punitive tone. They advocated that a psychiatrist consult with the primary physician and then participate conjointly in confronting the patient. The primary physician would inform the patient in a direct manner of the factitious diagnosis. The psychiatrist would help interpret to the patient that the factitious behavior was a cry for help. The physicians would attempt to reframe the disorder as a psychiatric one and encourage the patient to enter psychiatric treatment.

Psychiatrists began using this nonpunitive confrontation as the starting point of treatment, subsequently transferring the patient to inpatient psychiatric settings. Stone (1977) advocated involving family members to "close the circle" to prevent the patient from escaping psychiatric hospitalization, during which intensive psychotherapy was attempted. This technique had limited success. Stone's patient signed out of the psychiatric hospital against medical advice but later returned to outpatient treatment with another psychotherapist.

Some European psychiatrists (Hirsch 1994; Plassmann 1994b) have advocated a nonpunitive confrontation followed by an initial 2- to 6-month period of inpatient psychotherapy to build an alliance with the patient. The hospitalization is followed by several years of psychodynamically oriented therapy. Their work is of particular interest in terms of their understanding of the poorly regulated self-concepts that patients with factitious disorders commonly have. In addition, these authors have also speculated on the patient's use of his or her own body as a transitional object with an important security function for the individual. They have gone on to highlight the patient's tendency to develop negative therapeutic reactions caused by the often chaotic and hostile early developmental environment. These investigators report significant success with their psychodynamically oriented approach in 10 of 12 patients. Unfortunately, such lengthy treatments, particularly in inpatient settings, are not currently practical within the United States.

In the United States, some clinicians (Mayo and Haggerty 1984; Schoenfel et al. 1987; Tucker and Hayes 1979) have used nonpunitive confrontation to initiate long-term outpatient psychotherapy. These psychotherapy advocates generally incorporated a psychodynamically oriented approach, investigating the unconscious themes considered to be playing significant roles in the patient's behaviors. They often attempted to deal with illness episodes as metaphorical communications and had less concern with the origin of an illness. One group advocated educating the patient about the interpersonal communication involved in factitious behavior (Guziec et al. 1994). In their psychotherapy, they emphasize the theme "don't let your body do your talking," educating patients about how to express their feelings more adaptively.

Despite some success, however, confrontational approaches have had significant limitations. It is often difficult for a patient with factitious disorder to accept psychotherapy because this act may appear as an admission of the psychiatric origin. In many cases, confrontation does not accomplish much beyond driving the patient to seek care elsewhere. Clinicians have therefore been obliged to develop nonconfrontational strategies.

Nonconfrontational Strategies

A number of authors have described behavioral approaches to the treatment of factitious disorders. These approaches are less concerned with the origin of the illness and more concerned with shaping future behaviors.

Yassa (1978) reported the successful treatment of factitious behaviors in a patient using an operant conditioning paradigm during a state hospitalization spanning several years. Yassa developed a behavior modification program that rewarded acceptable social behavior with approval and praise while denying hospital privileges for pain complaints, acting out behavior, and feigned epileptic fits. In an outpatient setting, Klonoff et al. (1983–1984) applied a behavioral strategy to a patient with factitious nonepileptic seizures. This strategy involved positively reinforcing improvements while providing biofeedback as a face-saving vehicle for the patient's improvement. The face-saving aspect to the treatment is an important element that other behavioral approaches require as well. Without this aspect, it would be hard for patients to explain their recoveries without admitting that their prior detractors, who had claimed their problems were psychiatric, had been correct.

Solyom and Solyom (1990) developed a somewhat different behavioral approach for their two patients. Both patients had developed factitious paraplegia over several years. The Solyoms first confirmed the functional origin of the symptoms. After doing so, they specifically avoided commenting on the psychiatric origin of the disorder so the patients would not be required to increase their symptoms in order to prove their illnesses were genuinely organic. During the patients' hospitalizations, the staff avoided positively reinforcing any maladaptive behavior. They also added negative reinforcers for dysfunctional behavior. They told the patients that they would receive "faradic massage" with physiotherapy electrodes in order to "increase circulation and stimulate nerve endings." If their legs did not respond, the brief (1 to 6 minutes) but painful electrical massage duration would be increased. Both patients responded in less than 2 days, with significant leg movement, and they were ambulatory within 1 week. In order to "close the door" and prevent recurrence, the patients were videotaped in an ambulatory state. The rehabilitation plan also called for a single attending physician to follow the patients to provide continuity and forestall their attempts at rehospitalization. Utilizing this approach, the patients maintained their recovery over several-year periods, despite numerous emergency department visits involving efforts to be rehospitalized.

Schwartz and colleagues (1993) broadened the behavioral approach by devising a systems intervention for a patient with intractable factitious cellulitis. Their patient had a strong dependency on the hospital and had spent 235 days as an inpatient during the year prior to the intervention. Their innovative approach included the following: 1) paradoxical free access to the hospital with a designated permanent bed on a medical ward for 1 year; 2) the opportunity to enter or leave the hospital freely depending on the patient's own perceived need for treatment, without attempts at confrontation; 3) an emphasis on independent wound care assessment and decision making regarding the need for medical treatment; 4) a focus on holistic health and rehabilitation; 5) minimal consultation and radiologic and laboratory testing; 6) ongoing weekly psychotherapy with a primary care provider; and 7) amitriptyline for depressed mood. With this approach, the actual number of hospital days was reduced to 130 in the following year. Because the patient was charged for the room even when absent, the hospital charges were approximately 35% higher than the prior year. The charges were assumed by the hospital as indigent care and were not considered to represent a major financial loss because of low hospital census. Moreover, since her discharge, the patient had not been readmitted over a 16-month period. The approach altered the usual contingencies by not requiring the patient to manufacture disease in order to enter the hospital. By doing so, the patient's marked dependency needs were satisfied, apparently allowing her to move into a sustained recovery.

Eisendrath (1989, 1994, 1995) has recommended other behavioral strategies. He suggested that the face-saving aspect was critical to success, advocating techniques such as self-hypnosis ostensibly to enhance blood flow to a wound that had not healed. This intervention would allow the patient to have an acceptable rationale to explain his or her recovery. In one patient with whom this strategy was employed, the discussions about hypnosis also provided a safe vehicle for the patient to discuss emotionally charged issues that were difficult to discuss directly.

Another strategy that Eisendrath has advocated is the therapeutic double bind. In this approach, the patient is offered two choices: 1) prove that his or her disorder is not factitious by responding to a relatively minor and benign medical intervention; or 2) prove that the disorder is factitious by failing to respond. For example, one young woman was offered the double bind for a wound that had not healed in 4 years despite numerous surgical closures. Following the double bind strategy, the plastic surgeon told her that her wound should respond to a skin grafting procedure. If it did not, it would mean that her disorder was factitious in origin. This time the patient responded to the grafting by allowing the wound to heal.

Teasell and Shapiro (1994) utilized a double bind approach for rehabilitation patients with factitious motor disorders. They interpreted the patients' symptoms as due to a physical cause but amenable to full recovery. They then encouraged gradual increases in function through physical and occupational therapies. They also praised improvements in function and withdrew positive reinforcement for continuing signs of disability. Patients were told at the beginning of treatment that full recovery would indicate an organic etiology; less than complete recovery would indicate a psychiatric etiology to the disorder. The authors extended the range of the double bind by predicting, as discharge neared, that any relapse after discharge would indicate a psychiatric origin. Using this approach, Teasell and Shapiro achieved remarkable success in the three seriously impaired patients they described. Their strategy was successful in providing patients with a face-saving legitimization of both their illnesses and recoveries.

In a somewhat different attempt at permitting face-saving and engaging the patient in psychotherapy, Eisendrath (1989) advocated the use of inexact interpretations (Glover 1931). In this approach, the psychiatric consultant would give the patient a psychotherapeutic interpretation that was partially correct but incomplete. The interpretation would capture much of the psychodynamic formulation for the patient's behavior but stop short of overtly identifying the factitious origin. By avoiding overt confrontation about the factitious etiology, the consultant could help a patient avoid possible humiliation while making it safer for the patient to relinquish the symptom with a feeling of control.

In a number of these cases, the patients even revealed the factitious etiology, presumably because they felt they were not being forced to make the disclosures. For example, one woman was hospitalized for investigation and treatment of chronic abdominal pain that had been associated with several episodes of unexplained septicemia. She had been confronted at another hospital about the probable factitious nature of the septicemia and responded by changing physicians. During the medical evaluation, the psychiatric consultant learned that the septicemia had developed whenever she began to develop a sexual relationship with a man. She had a history of having been sexually abused by her father through the age of 15. While her medical evaluation was being carried out, her current boyfriend visited and proposed marriage to her. That evening she developed septicemia requiring intensive care. Medical investigation revealed no identifiable source of infection. The consultant suggested to her that she might have been feeling a need to punish herself whenever something good, such as the increased intimacy with her boyfriend, arose in her life. Within 2 days of exploring this theme, she spontaneously acknowledged that she had injected herself intravenously with a foreign substance to produce the septicemia. She entered outpatient psychotherapy and was successful in developing the ability to tolerate intimacy and eventually to marry.

Nonconfrontational strategies can be utilized when a factitious disorder is first diagnosed. They are also particularly useful when prior confrontations have failed to change the factitious behavior. There are, however, limits to these nonconfrontational approaches. For example, when some patients are diagnosed for the first time with a factitious disorder, it may be in the setting of a medical crisis. In one such case, a patient with aplastic anemia was currently hospitalized because of severe immunocompromise and thrombocytopenia when the factitious origin of her condition was revealed by a friend. Because of concerns that the patient was continuing surreptitiously to ingest bone marrow–suppressing chemotherapy drugs in the hospital, nonconfrontational approaches were avoided. The critical nature of her illness demanded an immediate confrontation by her physician and a request to search her room. Although the search did not reveal any chemotherapy agents, delay for a nonconfrontational approach could have had life-threatening consequences for this particular patient. Nonetheless, since many other cases of factitious physical disorder smolder for years, there is often an opportunity to attempt nonconfrontational techniques.

Countertransference

It is important for the clinician to be aware of his or her own countertransference concerning patients with factitious disorders. The manipulations and deceits these patients exercise may produce a sense of betrayal and anger in the caregiver (Feldman and Feldman 1995). In some instances, this anger leads the psychiatrist to become only a medical detective trying to catch the elusive villain.

Ideally, the psychiatrist will benefit from using countertransference feelings to enhance the understanding of the patient. For example, when one patient continued to generate factitious disease during a prolonged medical hospitalization, her psychotherapist began to feel helpless and unable to improve her condition. Once the psychotherapist became aware of the helpless feeling, he could better understand the patient's sense of herself growing up in a chaotic, physically abusive family. This awareness was then interpreted to the patient, who began to improve after the empathic connection was made. Willenberg (1994) has underscored the importance of understanding countertransference feelings of helplessness and frustration that patients with factitious disorder often generate.

The importance of a therapeutic relationship is revealed in the commentary of a recovering factitious disorder patient (M. Feldman, personal communication, January 1995). The patient noted that much of her factitious disorder stemmed from a need to obtain nurturance at any cost. She sought attention and support to fill "the empty void." She learned that medical crises were an excellent means to mobilize the medical care team to give her what she sought. She also learned that if a crisis did not exist, she would usually not receive much attention from her caregivers, thus activating the drive continually to create new crises. She noted that in order to recover, she needed to have someone who was interested in her as a person and not merely a collection of medical symptoms; in her case this was a minister. The minister listened to her life story and provided empathy.

Systems Interventions

Patient-oriented interventions as discussed previously are certainly crucial for altering the patient's behavior. No less important, however, are interventions aimed at the medical system when a factitious diagnosis is being considered by the medical caregivers (Eisendrath 1995). As discussed in Chapter 2, psychiatric consultation can often lead to improved diagnosis and earlier treatment. Once a diagnosis is made, the psychiatric consultant's role usually expands.

As noted in Chapter 10, it is natural for medical and nursing staffs to feel angry when the factitious diagnosis is made. The patient has deceived them and broken the social contract of the sick role that the patient is allowed to be in as long as he or she is also trying to get out of it. In addition, the patient has betrayed the honesty usually implicit in the physician-patient relationship. The psychiatric consultant can help staff members to ventilate and reduce the anger they feel when a factitious diagnosis is confirmed. If this step is not taken, the patient may suffer from inappropriate discharge or punitive decisions such as withholding of antibiotics.

These issues are often best addressed in a multidisciplinary staff meeting. The psychiatric consultant can help staff understand the likely psychodynamics underlying the factitious disorder. This education may also serve to diminish anger and allow staff to better care for the patient.

It is often useful to include ethicists, hospital attorneys, and risk management advisers in the multidisciplinary meeting. This forum allows for the development of practical intervention guidelines for the complex legal and ethical issues raised with factitious physical disorders. These issues include questions such as whether or not to obtain consent for room searches, or to reveal the diagnosis of the factitious disorder to referring physicians even when the patient refuses authorization (Ford and Abernathy 1991; Sadler 1987). These and other legal and ethical issues are discussed at greater length in Chapter 4.

Management Suggestions

Overall, certain management suggestions for factitious physical disorder patients emerge. Medical caregivers must maintain consistent and clear communication amongst themselves and with the patient. All care for the patient should be centralized at one hospital with one primary physician who coordinates and approves of any specialist consultation. Patients should not be allowed to split staff on a ward or individual physicians in the outpatient setting. They also need to have regular medical visits even if they have no active crises; similarly to strategies for somatization disorder (Kashner et al. 1992; Smith 1994), these regular visits tend to diminish the positive reinforcement of acute illness. They also allow the patient to receive nurturance and support when exhibiting "healthy" behaviors and reassure the patient that he or she will not be abandoned. Despite the patient's history of a factitious disorder, physicians should remain alert to the possibility of genuine organic illness (Feldman and Ford 1994; Gavin 1838). When comorbid psychiatric disorders are present, adjunctive medication may be of value (Folks 1995).

In factitious disorders, as in other psychiatric conditions, the overall aim of treatment is to replace maladaptive behaviors with healthier ones. For example, regular psychotherapy sessions represent a more adaptive way of receiving nurturance than repeated medical hospitalizations. Offering the patient a face-saving way to relinquish his or her factitious disorder is often critical to a strategic intervention. The goal of treatment is recovery, not confession.

As with other recovery processes, treating physicians should expect relapses during times of stress but not view them as permanent setbacks. Just as a psychiatrist should not feel that an alcoholic patient's "slip" is a personal failure, an exacerbation of factitious disorder should not be viewed nihilistically. Indeed, an exacerbation may represent a chance to learn more about the motivations driving the factitious behavior. In some instances, life experiences and general maturation will be necessary for the patient to recover. In those cases, one goal of treatment will be to help the patient limit the damage he or she self-induces in the interim. Physicians need to be aware of their countertransference; psychotherapists need to go further and use their countertransference to better understand the patient (Feldman and Feldman 1995).

Factitious Psychological Disorders

Factitious disorders with predominantly psychological signs and symptoms have been studied less thoroughly than factitious physical disorders (see Chapter 3). Most of the literature on factitious psychological disorders has focused on characterizing and understanding this phenomenon from both phenomenologic and psychodynamic perspectives, but has not addressed treatment strategies. This fact is not surprising, given the difficulties inherent in arriving at such a diagnosis in the first place. In addition, although patients with factitious psychological symptoms might initially seem more receptive to psychiatric treatment in that they have actively sought out psychiatrists, they actually seek them "on their own terms," as Gelenberg (1977) has pointed out. They want psychiatrists to believe their symptoms and are prone to leave treatment if the offer is made to treat their condition as a factitious one.

Before focusing on treatment, we must recognize that factitious psychological disorders represent a heterogeneous entity. Thus, a single-treatment approach will not work for all patients for three basic reasons: 1) there is a motivational continuum for symptom production from unconscious to fully conscious, and it may be very difficult to differentiate malingering from factitious symptoms (see Chapters 1 and 5); 2) the literature describes a vast array of different psychiatric symptoms and presentations, ranging from factitious psychosis (Pope et al. 1982) and factitious mourning (Phillips et al. 1983) to factitious alcohol abuse (Caradoc-Davies 1988), factitious posttraumatic stress disorder (Sparr and Pankratz 1983), and factitious eating disorders (Silber 1987).

Some patients oscillate among several factitious symptoms. More research is needed to delineate the phenomenology and significance of these different presentations, thus enabling the design of appropriate treatments; and 3) some patients present with both factitious physical and psychological symptoms. Treatment approaches may differ depending on which type of symptoms predominate. For example, treatment of factitious physical symptoms often centers on preventing further physical harm, whereas factitious psychological symptoms are not inherently harmful, with the exception of suicide gestures or attempts.

Just as with factitious physical disorders, of particular relevance for treatment is the differentiation of patients with long-standing abnormal illness behavior from patients who occasionally produce factitious psychological symptoms under acute stress. Illustrating the latter type of presentation, Silber (1987) reported "acquired pseudo eating disorder" in two adolescent girls coping with adjustment to hospitalization on a unit for serious medical conditions. One girl had multiple sclerosis, and the other had an intercurrent illness superimposed on paraplegic myelomeningocele. The patients developed or fabricated symptoms of an eating disorder after exposure to peers with true eating disorders who were hospitalized on the same unit. One patient refused food, lost weight, and claimed that she had self-induced vomiting when in fact she could not vomit. The other patient fabricated a past history of anorexia and bulimia and claimed that she had required a 1-year stay in a psychiatric hospital. The author conceptualized these symptoms as a "defense against a pervasive underlying depression" and a response to the "pressing need for peer acceptance." The first patient responded to the combination of a behavior-modification protocol, an antidepressant, and psychotherapeutic counseling. She regained her weight, and her acquired pseudo eating disorder resolved. The second patient eventually acknowledged having devised her story "as a way of capturing her peers' attention and interest." She subsequently suffered an episode of depression but refused psychiatric intervention. However, her acquired pseudo eating disorder did not recur during a 1-year follow-up. In these patients, the acuity of their factitious symptoms appeared to have had favorable prognostic implications.

At the other end of the spectrum are patients with long-standing factitious psychological disorders, who, given the chronicity of their abnormal behavior, meet criteria for the diagnosis of Munchausen syndrome. These patients may present with factitious psychotic symptoms, depressive symptoms, posttraumatic stress symptoms, or a mixture of them all. Pope and colleagues (1982) identified a cohort of nine patients with factitious psychosis from among 219 patients consecutively admitted to a psychiatric research ward. Although their article focuses on phenomenology and family history, some of their observations are relevant for treatment. For example, they found a high incidence of comorbid personality disorders and substance abuse, which must be considered in the management of these patients. The authors found their patients to have a very poor long-term outcome at 4- to 6-year follow-up. Several patients who were excluded from their selected cohort of nine appeared to display both real and factitious psychotic symptoms "in the same manner that factitious seizures are often seen in patients who also have true epilepsy." As suggested elsewhere by Popli and colleagues (1992), psychological symptoms may be exposed as factitious when they fail to respond to several effective medications or respond to medications not expected to be helpful. However, the presence of factitious symptoms does not exclude the need for antipsychotic medication for concurrent true psychosis. In these cases, accurate diagnosis is essential for treatment, and psychological testing may aid in diagnosis.

Emphasis on a different kind of factitious psychological disorder is illustrated by two series of patients presenting with themes related to loss. In one report, Snowdon and associates (1978) raised the possibility of underlying true depressive symptomatology in 11 of 12 cases of feigned bereavement. Phillips and colleagues (1983) reported 20 patients with factitious mourning and also pointed out the possibility of underlying genuine depression. Both papers stressed the importance of understanding the patients' true feelings. The authors also suggested that the patients may have suffered genuine losses, even though these may have been different from the ones they reported. For example, Snowdon and colleagues (1978) reported the case of a 42-year-old man who claimed that his wife and daughter had just been killed. In fact, they were still alive, but the patient had actually been divorced by two wives. Many of these patients are thought to use their factitious symptoms as a way of feeling in control rather than facing a loss that might be overwhelming.

The previous authors' recommendations for management are limited and based on experience during inpatient treatment, not outpatient care. Snowdon and colleagues (1978) emphasized attempting to understand why the stories were being told. They also stressed the importance of discussion among inpatient staff members in order to deal with countertransference feelings and avoid a tendency to punish these patients. Phillips and associates (1983) supported patient confrontation—a controversial approach to treatment, as mentioned above—in order to reduce staff resentment and "curtail development of pathological careers" in these patients. They also recommended referral to outpatient therapy whenever possible to encourage the patients to work on characterologic issues. The literature has not addressed the question of whether using antidepressant medication would help factitious mourning patients with suspected underlying major depression, but such an effect appears likely.

A unique case report by Parker (1993) illustrates some of the challenges of ongoing outpatient treatment. This is the only case report in the literature describing long-term treatment of a patient with factitious psychological disorder. The case involved a 51-year-old woman who initially presented with symptoms of delirium and claimed that she had been beaten and raped 1 month prior to admission. In the hospital, her illness was managed as a conversion symptom. A nonconfrontational approach was used, consisting of acknowledging to the patient that she had been through a very difficult experience while reassuring her that she would get better. The patient's symptoms gradually improved over 2 weeks. Shortly after discharge, the patient was lost to follow-up until 8 months later, when she asked for an appointment and was subsequently treated for 8 months in outpatient psychotherapy.

The therapist initially focused on limit-setting, especially regarding the patient's being on time for appointments, and she determined that weekly 30-minute sessions were optimal for this patient's abilities to interact with the therapist. Attention-seeking behaviors were ignored, and therapy was informed by a nonconfrontational approach. Though the alleged assault and rape had probably been fabricated, there was strong evidence of a history of sexual abuse.

This case seems to point to the importance of paying attention to the affective tone to the factitious history, though the actual facts may not be true. As expressed by Gelenberg (1977) in his case report of a patient with factitious psychological disorder, the patient's "complaints seemed closer to the bedrock of unconscious pain, his expressed wishes for psychiatric treatment nearer to his true needs." Just as with other material such as dreams, factitious psychological symptoms may guide the psychotherapist in understanding the patient's emotional life.

Conclusion

Factitious disorders represent massive challenges for the treating clinician. As we have attempted to demonstrate, however, effective interventions are possible. These approaches require the clinician's flexibility and creativity. Further development of successful treatment strategies for factitious disorders will rest on a clearer understanding of their phenomenology and psychodynamics. Attention to comorbidity with other psychiatric conditions, particularly for factitious psychological disorders, may yield more information on potential treatment approaches.

Thus, we conclude that the therapeutic nihilism associated with the subset of patients with Munchausen syndrome appears inappropriate for the vast majority of factitious disorder patients.

References

Asher R: Munchausen's syndrome. Lancet 1:339–341, 1951

Birch CA: Munchausen's syndrome. Lancet 1:412, 1951

Caradoc-Davies G: Feigned alcohol abuse: a unique case report. Br J Psychiatry 152:418–420, 1988

Cohen LM, Shapiro E, Manson JE, et al: The high cost of treating a psychiatric disorder as a medical/surgical illness. Psychosomatics 26:453–455, 1985

Earle JR, Folks DG: Factitious disorder and coexisting depression: a report of successful psychiatric consultation and case management. Gen Hosp Psychiatry 8:448–450, 1986

Eisendrath SJ: Factitious physical disorders: treatment without confrontation. Psychosomatics 30:383–387, 1989

Eisendrath SJ: Factitious physical disorders. West J Med 160:177–179, 1994

Eisendrath SJ: Factitious disorders and malingering, in Treatments of Psychiatric Disorders: The DSM-IV Edition. Edited by Gabbard GO. Washington, DC, American Psychiatric Press, 1995

Feldman MD: The costs of factitious disorders. Psychosomatics 35:506–507, 1994

Feldman MD, Feldman JM: Tangled in the web: countertransference in the therapy of factitious disorders. Int J Psychiatry Med 25:379–389, 1995

Feldman MD, Ford CV: Patient or Pretender: Inside the Strange World of Factitious Disorders. New York, Wiley, 1994, pp 107–117

Folks DG: Munchausen's syndrome and other factitious disorders. Neurol Clin 13:267–281, 1995

Folks DG, Houck CA: Somatoform disorders, factitious disorders, and malingering, in Psychiatric Care of the Medical Patient. Edited by Stoudemire A, Fogel B. New York, Oxford University Press, 1993, pp 267–287

Ford CV, Abernethy V: Factitious illness: a multidisciplinary consideration of ethical issues. Gen Hosp Psychiatry 3:329–336, 1981

Fras I, Coughlin BE: Treatment of factitious disease. Psychosomatics 12:117–122, 1971

Gavin H: On Feigned and Factitious Diseases. Edinburgh, University Press, 1838, pp 27–28

Gelenberg AJ: Munchausen's syndrome with a psychiatric presentation. Diseases of the Nervous System 38:378–380, 1977

Geracioti TD, Van Dyke C, Mueller J, et al: The onset of Munchausen's syndrome. Gen Hosp Psychiatry 9:405–409, 1987

Glover E: Therapeutic effect of inexact interpretation: a contribution to the theory of suggestion. Int J Psychoanal 12:397–411, 1931

Guziec DO, Lazarus A, Harding JJ: Case of a 29-year-old nurse with factitious disorder: the utility of psychiatric intervention on a general medical floor. Gen Hosp Psychiatry 16:47–53, 1994

Hirsch M: The body as a transitional object. Psychother Psychosom 62:78–81, 1994

Hollender MD, Hersh SR: Impossible consultation made possible. Arch Gen Psychiatry 23:343–345, 1970

Ifudu O, Kolasinski SL, Friedman EA: Kidney-related Munchausen's syndrome. N Engl J Med 327:388–389, 1992

Kashner TM, Rost K, Smith GR, et al: An analysis of panel data: the impact of a psychiatric consultation letter on the expenditures and outcomes of care for patients with somatization disorder. Medical Care 30:811–821, 1992

Klonoff EA, Youngner SJ, Moore DJ, et al: Chronic factitious illness: a behavioral approach. Int J Psychiatry Med 13:73–83, 1983–1984

Mayo JP, Haggerty JJ: Long-term therapy of Munchausen syndrome. Am J Psychother 38:571–578, 1984

McElroy SL, Phillips KA, Keck PE Jr.: Obsessive compulsive spectrum disorder. J Clin Psychiatry 55:33–51, 1994

Menninger KA: Polysurgery and polysurgical addiction. Psychoanal Q 3:173–199, 1934

Parker PE: A case report of Munchausen syndrome with mixed psychological features. Psychosomatics 34:360–364, 1993

Phillips MR, Ward NG, Ries RK: Factitious mourning: painless patienthood. Am J Psychiatry 140:420–425, 1983

Plassmann R: The biography of the factitious-disorder patient. Psychother Psychosom 62:123–128, 1994a

Plassmann R: Inpatient and outpatient long-term psychotherapy of patients suffering from factitious disorders. Psychother Psychosom 62:96–107, 1994b

Pope HG, Jonas JM, Jones B: Factitious psychosis: phenomenology, family history, and long-term outcome of nine patients. Am J Psychiatry 139:1480–1483, 1982

Popli AP, Masand PS, Dewan MJ: Factitious disorders with psychological symptoms. J Clin Psychiatry 53:315–318, 1992

Powell R, Boast N: The Million Dollar Man: resource implications for chronic Munchausen's syndrome. Br J Psychiatry 162:253–256, 1993

Rasmussen SA: Obsessive compulsive spectrum disorders. J Clin Psychiatry 55:89–91, 1994

Sadler JZ: Ethical and management considerations in factitious illness: one and the same. Gen Hosp Psychiatry 9:31–39, 1987

Schoenfel H, Margolin J, Baum S: Munchausen syndrome as a suicide equivalent: abolition of syndrome by psychotherapy. Am J Psychother 41:604–612, 1987

Schwartz K, Harding R, Harrington D, et al: Hospital management of a patient with intractable factitious disorder. Psychosomatics 34:265–267, 1993

Silber TJ: Acquired pseudo eating disorder: an imitation or fabrication of anorexia nervosa. J Adolesc Health Care 8:452–455, 1987

Smith GR: The course of somatization and its effects on utilization of health care resources. Psychosomatics 35:263–267, 1994

Snowdon J, Solomons R, Druce H: Feigned bereavement: twelve cases. Br J Psychiatry 133:15–19, 1978

Solyom C, Solyom L: A treatment program for functional paraplegia/Munchausen syndrome. J Behav Ther Exp Psychiatry 21:225–230, 1990

Sparr L, Pankratz LD: Factitious posttraumatic stress disorder. Am J Psychiatry 140:1016–1019, 1983

Stone MH: Factitious illness: psychological findings and treatment recommendations. Bull Menninger Clin 41:239–254, 1977

Teasell RW, Shapiro AP: Strategic-behavioral intervention in the treatment of chronic nonorganic motor disorders. Am J Phys Med Rehabil 73:44–50, 1994

Tucker LE, Hayes JR: Factitial bleeding: successful management with psychotherapy. Dig Dis Sci 24:570–572, 1979

Van Moffaert M: Management of self-mutilation. Psychother Psychosom 51:180–186, 1989

Willenberg H: Countertransference in factitious disorder. Psychother Psychosom 62:129–134, 1994

Yassa R: Munchausen's syndrome: a successfully treated case. Psychosomatics 19:242–243, 1978

Index

Page numbers printed in **boldface** *type refer to tables or figures.*